Medical Ethics in the Renaissance

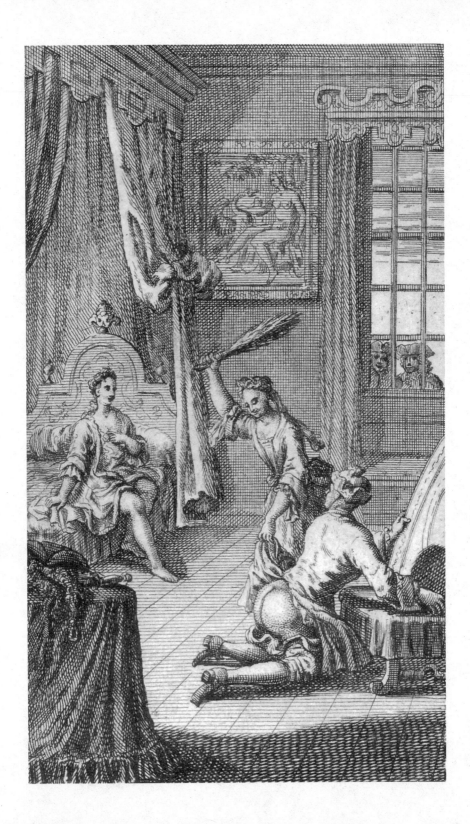

Medical Ethics in the Renaissance

Winfried Schleiner

GEORGETOWN UNIVERSITY PRESS / WASHINGTON, D.C.

Georgetown University Press, Washington, D.C.   20007
© 1995 by Georgetown University Press. All rights reserved.
Printed in the United States of America.
10 9 8 7 6 5 4 3 2 1   1995
THIS VOLUME IS PRINTED ON ACID-FREE OFFSET BOOKPAPER.

Library of Congress Cataloging-in-Publication Data

Schleiner, Winfried.
    Medical ethics in the Renaissance   /   Winfried Schleiner.
        p.   cm.
    Includes bibliographical references.
    1. Medicine—Europe—History—15th century.   2. Medicine—Europe—
History—16th century.   3. Medicine—Europe—History—17th century.
I. Title.
R724.S3934   1995
174′.2′09—dc20
ISBN 0-87840-593-3

                                                                    95-7359

Contents

Introduction

If it did not sound pretentious and smack of reverse modesty, I would call this study "Prolegomena to Renaissance Medical Ethics." It represents the efforts of a person who has read widely, if not wisely, at some of the best libraries for this subject in the United States and Europe. In view of the immense range of the medical literature of the Renaissance, certain choices and exclusions had to be made, some on principle, others by practical necessity. The latter may be defended with an adage ascribed to Hippocrates: *ars longa, vita brevis*. Since this study covers the period (from about the mid-sixteenth to about the mid-seventeenth century) in which, toward the end, something like a self-conscious field of medical ethics constitutes itself, many of the earlier works treated may represent an "archaeology" of medical ethics. Roughly, then, the period of my interest starts with the high point of medical humanism (as Nancy Siraisi has defined it) and ends with the gradual replacement or passing out of favor of Aristotelian natural philosophy and Galenic physiology.[1]

It would not have aided my study to start with any limiting and necessarily debatable definition of what I thought this field to be, although for merely heuristic purposes I have considered medical ethics an ethics of medical doctors. Obvious or even commonsensical as it may seem, this decision had many consequences, most of them welcome, because they narrowed my field: I am not, except for an occasional aside (justified usually by a physician's reference), writing about the moral casuistry of theologians, although I recognize that they, too, frequently discuss medical questions and even sometimes the same questions as the physicians. That field alone is so immense that, although my interest in it had been kindled by such fine work as that by Amundsen and Noonan,[2] I was not sorry to leave it aside. An imaginative reader will have to add it, however, to complement and complete the picture, because many physicians in the period, and arguably the best thinkers on medical ethics, were very much aware of it. Indeed, the Protestant Heinrich Meibom, writing in Protestant Lübeck, is proof that intimate knowledge of Roman Catholic moral casuistry (and the various papal pronouncements on issues relating to health and medicine) was not limited to Catholic physicians. Another decision, forced upon me and less justifiable by the "matter" itself, was the exclusion of Paracelsian and alchemical medicine, which has attracted some of the most probing modern attention. But since I had to set limits somehow and limit the scope of my work, it made sense to concentrate on what in the period was called "rational" medicine by its proponents, the medicine in the Hippocratic-Galenic tradition taught at, and unquestionably dominating, most European universities.

Even within the area thus circumscribed, which is still vast, certain choices had to be made. In some sense, much medical thinking in the Renaissance is commentary on the ancients, not always respectful and even sometimes quite acerbic—whether Abraham Zacuto writes, as it were, a variorum edition of commentary on established medical cases and Mercuriale, the famous professor at Padua, Bologna, and finally at Pisa, squeezes Hippocratic case histories until his readings exceed the originals by a ratio of thirty to one,[3] or whether the work of a *neotericus*, though structured independently and differently, yet refers to the ancient physicians at every step. Therefore one might make a case for beginning each chapter and section of a study like mine with Hippocrates and Galen or at least with delineating in detail the ancient medical tradition. This might have resulted in a more scholarly seeming study. But some matters discussed at considerable length in these pages simply were not clearly conceptualized by the ancient physicians or not conceptualized in a way that was helpful to the Renaissance. The matter of pretense in curing is one example; possibly the seam or line between or (as we might fashionably say) the interface between medical and religious duties is another—although there were ancient comments on the latter, as when, according to a passage in the Hippocratic corpus, medicine because of its limited powers treats the gods "in most cases" with reverence.[4] Another and tempting alternative approach I could have adopted would have been to structure my study around Renaissance commentaries on the "Hippocratic" oath. But even the learned Meibom in his commentary on that text admits that of the seven Renaissance commentaries of which he knows, he has not been able to lay hands on two. I was not confident that I could do better. More important, however revealing such a comparison might be, it would have limited my approach significantly, and I could not have ventured an opinion on most of the matters at the center of this study.

Our knowledge of Renaissance medical ethics is quite limited, even though curing in the period was strongly informed by an ethical sense and physicians expressed their ethical motives in writing (and in print), because there are few whole works devoted mostly or in considerable portions to what we might call medical ethics. I hope I have included the handful that are: books by Alexandrinus, Bardi, Botallo, Rodrigo a Castro, Fidele, Fontecha, Henriques, Meibomius, Moxius (or Moix), and Ranchin. That from other perspectives than mine the work I use from a writer like Fontecha (it is an introductory text for medical students) may be of minor significance is no argument against highlighting it in my context, because it is full of observations about a physician's moral conduct and ways of resolving a moral dilemma. In some respect, the history of medicine has to be rethought from the perspective of medical ethics. This would be brought home most clearly if readers of this volume were to check on some of the names mentioned above in the still extremely useful biographical dictionary by August Hirsch. Meibomius, they would find, for instance, "wrote only insignificant works."[5] It is clear that in an earlier period the history of medicine has often been biased in favor of medicine as a presumably objective science. Even those few names listed here have to my knowledge never been assembled, although some of them have their place in histories of forensic medicine (like Esther Fischer Homberger's).[6] It may be indicative of the general lack of modern bibliographic aids for work in medical ethics of this period that the multivolume catalogue of the medical and scientific holdings of the Herzog August Bibliothek, Wolfenbüttel, generally an indispensable tool for a thematic access to the field of Renaissance medicine, has no entry for "Ethik." Of course I came upon the works of the authors listed above gradually, and I am not confident that I have discovered all those with a concern for medical ethics.

In general, I have used two kinds of pilots through this sea of medical books. First, I have been led by the Renaissance physicians themselves, as, for example, the chapter on what a physician's library should contain in Rodrigo a Castro's *Medicus-Politicus* (lib. 2, c. 9), although one problem is (as I will argue later) that the author may be leaving out some important books rather deliberately. Second, toward the end or closure of the period of my concern, there are, fortunately, such encyclopedic works as Zacchia's and Boudewyn's, which can be used as guides specifically in medical ethics and forensic medicine, pointing to what was considered important in the Renaissance. Naturally they also have their biases.

Ultimately, however, to get some impression of how any ethical problem was conceived, we have to go to a variety of works presenting medical *quaestiones, disputationes, casus, curationes, observationes, consilia, epistolae*, etc. For serendipitous finds of texts indicating a physician's bafflement, confusion, moral dilemmas (including some that introduce my chapters), nothing is so rewarding and pleasurable as reading medical works according to a shelf list in a good library. For that reason, many names are mentioned in this study, and because of its physical constraints I have not always been able to indicate the historical or intellectual context to which they belong. While the plethora of little-known names may complicate reading these chapters, I am strongly convinced that for the goals I set myself, a comparative reading ranging broadly over works from authors of different countries and different beliefs leads to more insights than one that would narrow the focus to one place or year. Another consequence of reading Renaissance medical works by shelf lists will be obvious to anyone familiar with the vastness of the field: there really is no end or closure to this kind of study, for there is always another library with more and different books.

Finally, although this study is based on patient perusal of old texts, I am very conscious of my own biases and interests. A topic like the role of pretense in medicine (chapter 2) is perhaps chosen over others primarily because feigning and make-believe have been at the core of theories of imaginative literature; a topic like the removal of male and female seed, in chapter 5 (the latter part treating the history of hysteria), relates to the modern interest in the construction of gender and sexuality, a field in which some of the most exciting historical and literary work is being conducted at present; and in the background of my interest in syphilis (chapter 6), which was then considered by most physicians a new disease, are modern discussions of the construction of disease and particularly debates about how far one should go in the prevention of AIDS.

NOTES

1. See Nancy G. Siraisi, *Avicenna in Renaissance Italy: The Canon and Medical Teaching in Italian Universities after 1500* (Princeton, N.J.: Princeton University Press, 1987), particularly pp. 64–65 and 120. On the undermining of Galenic physiology, see Owsei Temkin, *Galenism: Rise and Decline of a Medical Philosophy* (Ithaca, N.Y.: Cornell University Press, 1973), p. 161. Charles B. Schmitt has demonstrated how important Aristotle continued to be throughout the Renaissance and writes of "the vast subject of translations of the 'Nicomachean Ethics' in the sixteenth century." See "Aristotle's Ethics in the Sixteenth Century: Some Preliminary Considerations," in Schmitt, *The Aristotelian Tradition and Renaissance Universities* (London: Variorum Reprints, 1984), essay VII, p. 91.

2. See, for example, Darrel W. Amundsen, "Casuistry and Professional Obligations: The Regulation of Physicians by the Court of Conscience in the Late Middle Ages (Part I)" and "Casuistry and Professional Obligations: The Regulation of Physicians by the Court of Conscience in the Late Middle Ages (Part II)," *Transactions and Studies of the College of Physicians of Philadelphia*, 5th ser., vol. 3 (1981): pp. 22–29 and 93–112 and John T. Noonan, *Contraception: A History of Its Treatment by the Catholic Theologians and Canonists* (Cambridge, Mass.: Harvard University Press, 1986).

3. Mercuriale, *Pisanae praelectiones. In Epidemicas Hippocratis historias* (Venice, 1597).

4. *Peri euschemosynes (De habitu medicinae ad religionem)*, in Hippocrates, *Oeuvres complètes*, ed. Emile Littré, vol. 9, p. 235: "Pour l'ensemble des maladies et des symptômes, la médecine est, dans la plupart des cas, pleine de révérence à l'égard des dieux. Devant les dieux les médecins s'inclinent, car la médecine n'a pas une puissance qui surabonde." On the relationship between Hippocratic medicine and early Christianity, see Owsei Temkin, *Hippocrates in a World of Pagans and Christians* (Baltimore and London: Johns Hopkins University Press, 1991). Owsei Temkin has also described some of the reactions of Jewish, Christian, and Muslim theologians to Galen's professed agnosticism. See Temkin, *Galenism: Rise and Decline of a Medical Philosophy*, particularly p. 92.

5. Hirsch, *Biographisches Lexikon der hervorragenden Ärzte aller Zeiten*, 2d ed. (Berlin and Wien: Urban and Schwarzenberg, 1932): "Er schrieb nur unbedeutende Schriften." It should be noted, however, that this work largely records views of the 1880s, when the first edition appeared.

6. E. Fischer Homberger, *Medizin vor Gericht: Gerichtsmedizin von der Renaissance bis zur Aufklärung* (Bern, Stuttgart, Wien: Huber, 1983).

Acknowledgments

Two fellowships enabled me to do concentrated work at crucial periods of this project: a University of California President's Research Fellowship in the Humanities (1989–90) and a National Endowment for the Humanities/Folger Shakespeare Library Fellowship (1991–92). I thank my institution, the University of California, Davis, for funds (administered by the UC Davis Committee on Research and the UC Davis Washington Center) supporting repeated trips to the National Library of Medicine, the Folger Shakespeare Library, and the Huntington Library. I am grateful to Ms. Susan Kancir for typing the manuscript. Publication was supported by a publication subsidy from the University of California, Davis (from the College of Letters and Science and from the Office of Research) and a mini-grant from the Andrew W. Mellon Publication Endowment at the Folger Shakespeare Library.

Material published in three articles appears here in different guise and context: a segment of chapter 3 was published in *The Expulsion of the Jews: 1492 and After,* ed. R. B. Waddington and A. H. Williamson and portions of chapter 4 appeared in *The Bulletin of the History of Medicine* and *The Journal of Medieval and Renaissance Studies.* I am grateful to these publishers for their permission to reuse this material. This book on a medical literature written primarily in what Francis Bacon called "the universal language" could not have been completed without occasional but crucial help by colleagues more versed in that language than I: Lynn Roller, David Traill, and Peter M. Schaeffer at the University of California, Davis, and Patricia Harris-Stäblein at the Folger Library. At a time when the viability of programs in classics is being questioned at my institution and elsewhere, this service to me, which will not show up in student counts, needs to emphasized.

Scholars who gave me encouragement at moments when the project seemed to falter include James H. Cassedy (National Library of Medicine), Werner Gundersheimer (Folger Library), Barbara K. Lewalski (Harvard University), Everett Carter (University of California, Davis), Stephen Greenblatt (Harvard University), and above all my wife, Louise (Washington State University), who in spite of her own busy schedule has remained my most careful reader. This book may also be an answer to my daughter Christa, who in our constricted living quarters in Cambridge, England, when the dining room table had become my study, noted that it "looked ugly."

Medical Ethics in the Renaissance

1

Ethics: Some Preliminary Reflections

When Renaissance physicians recommend one particular text on ethics to their students, it is usually Aristotle's *Nichomachean Ethics*.[1] Charles B. Schmitt has said that this book "as much as any work from antiquity, emerged from the Reformation struggles as a keystone of both Catholic and Protestant education."[2] But thinking on the subject of ethics in the period is more than just commenting on that text. As an example of what students were told at a major (Protestant) university that produced many a "rational" physician, it may be useful to begin by looking at Melanchthon's influential book on moral philosophy (*Philosophia moralis Epitomes*, Strassburg, 1542). I am aware, of course, that at present I am following only one thread of an intricate web, for in Roman Catholic countries moral casuistry (which, as such, has an obvious proximity to and usefulness for medical casuistry, and derives, as the practitioners often reveal by their references to *canonistae et summistae*, principally from canon law and Thomas Aquinas's *Summa*) was soon to blossom to extraordinary heights. According to Melanchthon, ethics is a *lex* or *ius naturae*, a natural law supporting right reason (*recta ratio*). If I add, as I must, that according to him this "natural law" is also "divine law" (*lex divina*), modern readers may question the usefulness of such distinction: it may seem meaningless to collapse "natural" and "divine." Melanchthon's distinctions are made in the Thomistic tradition, many features of which outlasted the Reformation. The important point is that Melanchthon excludes revelation through the New Testament from right reason as supported by natural (or divine) law. He repeatedly insists on the crucial difference between these two sources of knowledge and encourages his reader to check how far the principles derived from them overlap—ultimately he considers them complementary. Several years later, in *Ethicae doctrinae elementa* (Wittenberg, 1550), he clarified the matter by saying that by "law" he intended the knowledge (*doctrina*) with which God endowed human minds in the creation (p. 4). For my later discussion of the book on medical ethics by Rodrigo a Castro, *Medicus-Politicus* (Hamburg 1614), a book drawing frequently on examples from the Old Testament, it will be important to remember that in Melanchthon's distinction the Old Testament with its decalogue forms part of *philosophia moralis* and thus is part of general ethics—only the New Testament with its message of forgiveness and grace is part of revelation.

To understand Melanchthon's thinking about ethics, we also need to see that by natural law (*ius naturae*), the subject of ethics, he understands practical principles and observations about outward actions: "The law of nature signifies the natural ideas about practices, i.e. practical principles and right conclusions and necessary consequences arising from those principles."[3] From the modern point of view, i.e. after the Kantian revolution in ethics (Kant, by contrast, made precisely the inner motivations the subject of ethics—although in his famous categorical imperative he connected inner motivation with duties applying to all humanity), this insistence on the practical and exterior may seem striking,[4] but it brings us closer to the subject of medicine. After all, the question whether medicine was one of the *artes* or whether it was *scientia* (was it theoretical, or a more menial skill or craft?) was often discussed in the Renaissance. Heinrich Lavater, for instance, decided that medicine was neither, properly speaking (*proprie*), but if one had to classify it, he suggested classifying it with the *artes*; and the frontispiece of Giovanni Battista Cortesi's *Miscellaneorum medicinalium decades* (which will occupy us later; see figure 5.3) frames the title between the allegorical figures of *ratio* and *experientia*.

For Melanchthon the practical and civil usefulness of ethics has to do with the certainty it affords all human beings, and it is interesting that for him in this context (moral) philosophy, i.e. ethics, and medicine are connected: "One should reject those academics who withhold from the arts the praise of certainty, notwithstanding that thus medicine and [moral] philosophy deal with probable relations whose degree of certainty is up to the practicioner [of those arts] to judge. For that which conflicts with principles is to be rejected right away."[5] Melanchthon's emphasis not only moves ethics to the practical, civil (and possibly public) side, it also legitimizes the study of pagan ethics (including the ethical thinking of ancient physicians) as something useful.

Very much in the Protestant tradition, the German Theophilus Golius (1528–1600), whose influential work on ethics was also printed in Cambridge, finds that an ethics thus defined, namely as principles about "outward" habits and actions, is extremely useful in civil life, and advocates studying the pagan philosophers. However he adds an important proviso that in fact brings Protestant speculation about ethics close to the Catholic/Thomistic strain: the ethical teachings of pagan philosophers ought to be retained as useful "on the condition that divine or Christian ethics shines forth as ruler (*domina*) and has precedence while profane and philosophical ethics follows as if she were her apprentice and servant (*famula et ministra*) and is directed (*regatur*) by her light."[6] I must leave to the Reformation historians to answer the question whether this hierarchy was already implied by Melanchthon though not made explicit, or whether it is an expression of the generally more repressive tendencies of the reformers of the second and third generation, concerned with ecclesiastical uniformity.

Beyond the insistence on the practical nature of ethics (which Golius retains from Melanchthon's thinking), it may seem that this position might not differ sufficiently from Catholic ethics to result in significantly different moral decisions when applied to *praxis*, for instance that of a physician. What is important, however, is that the differentiation of the two modes of knowledge (natural or philosophical versus revealed) is one of the most basic distinctions Protestant thinkers on ethics make. (Melanchthon and Golius make it on the first few pages of their influential books.) While the hierarchy between the moral "institutions" (of ruler and ruled) is clearly outlined, the insistence on a clear dividing line, a difference, was important. It provided Protestant readers, including the medical students to whom Melanchthon lectured at Wittenberg, with the intellectual teeth, the categories or demarcations, to reflect on their own experience. Also it is true that once such a distinction between areas of knowledge became established, their hierarchy could be called into question and eventually even be turned upside down.

Before I rush ahead too far, however, I need to point out that the distinction between "philosophical ethics" and "Christian ethics" is only analogous to, and not identical with, the various binary distinctions that I find Renaissance physicians of all persuasions are beginning to make as they halt and analyze, justify or defend their own actions, or evaluate, criticize, and even attack someone else's. For they oppose the duties of the physician to those of the clergyman, the treatment of the body to the treatment of the soul; they say "we Christians" as different from others; and they make a distinction between a question that is medical and one that is theological. Most of these distinctions serve to arrogate responsibility from the clergy to the doctors, and thus may be one aspect of a growing secularization of European culture, which is, however, far from continous and ubiquitous (unlike the proverbial rise of the middle class); and since this is done in print and usually in the still international medium of the Latin language, the phenomenon is also part of the growing public area or space, or *Öffentlichkeit*, to use Jürgen Habermas's term.

NOTES

1. See, for example, Hippolitus Obicius, *De nobilitate medici contra illius obtrectatores. Dialogus tripartitus* (Venice, 1606), pp. 206–10.

2. Schmitt, "Aristotle's Ethics in the Sixteenth Century: Some Preliminary Considerations," in his *The Aristotelian Tradition and Renaissance Universities* (London: Variorum Reprints, 1984): item VII, p. 94.

3. *Ethicae doctrinae elementa*, p. 80: "Ius naturae significat naturales noticias de moribus, hoc est, principia practica et conclusiones recta et necessaria consequentia ex illis orta."

4. For a fine summary of the larger contexts, see the entry "Ethik" in *Historisches Wörterbuch der Philosophie* (Basel und Stuttgart: Schwabe, 1971–[1992]), vol. 2, particularly col. 783.

5. *Philosophia moralis epitomes*, p. 4: "Sunt igitur explodendi Academici, qui artibus detrahunt laudem certitudinis, verum ut medicina et philosophia assumit interdum probabiles relationes, quae quatenus valeant, artificis est iudicare; Nam illa quae pugnant cum principiis prorsus repudianda sunt."

6. Golius, *Epitome doctrina moralis, ex decem libris Ethicorum Aristotelis ad Nicomachum collecta* (Cambridge, 1634), p. 3.

2

Mentiamur sane:
Lying for Health in
Renaissance Medical Ethics

In what has been called the first book on forensic medicine, the Sicilian physician Fortunato Fidele (1550–1630) tells the following case:

> I knew a girl in her flourishing youth, who consulted her physician about aborting a fetus before its time. In order to foil her undertaking, the physician, in a pious misrepresentation (*pia simulatione*), promised her he would give her something that would fulfill her expectation entirely: but in truth he mixed an antidote from ingredients that should make the fetus strong and healthy. However, the girl had hardly drunk it down, when she began to burn with the desire to bring forth, and hoping that what she had been promised falsely would certainly happen, entirely bent on this one concern, she before long felt the fetus had dropped down; and to the disgrace (*ignominia*) of the physician, she aborted in spite of the resisting medication. For the image of the abortion, so strongly conceived, both overcame the power of the medication and foiled the physician's endeavor.[1]

Fidele's rather bare account illustrates the nexus of a number of threads that this chapter will untangle. Thus my discussion can be thought of as one giant footnote on this brief report, to which I intend to return at the end of the chapter.

If the question whether medical deception is permitted in the interest of cure has been selected here as a way into the subject of medical ethics, the reason is not that I would want to suggest that premodern physicians were pseudoscientists or that the discipline might have been tormented by self-doubt or the suspicion of fakery, although such encompassing doubt about Hippocratic/Galenic medicine is common in opposing camps and is occasionally voiced on the fringes of the discipline. Thus Antonio Carera (fl. 1652) reports that one of his professors at Padua once defined the art of medicine as "the art of deceiving the world, by which the entire world is deceived."[2] Perhaps there is, in this indictment, a memory of Hippocrates comparing bad physicians to actors on the stage, who are only masks (*personae* in the Latin translation) of physicians.[3] Both in the Hippocratic corpus and in Galen, there are occasionally references to deception in curing (the practical need to conceal the unpleasantness of prescriptions, i.e. "sugar-coating," and the equally practical and forensic need to detect people simulating illness are examples), but deception is not really conceived as an important theoretical issue. One indication, if not proof, of this is that when in the Renaissance Rodrigo a Castro in his *Medicus-Politicus* sets out to raise some fundamental questions about this issue and starts, as is his wont, with a scheme of opposing classical authorities on the subject, he does not use medical authorities, but Plato and Aristotle—all the ancient physicians are on one side in this matter. While it is sometimes tempting to consider Renaissance medicine a seamless continuation of and even mere commentary on, ancient medical thinking, Renaissance medical interest in deception is one of no doubt many topics calling into question such a commonplace.

I have selected the complex of problems relating to truth and falsehood for a number of reasons that will become obvious, but at this point I would alert the reader to four: (1) In the subsequent history of ethics, the dispute over the question of whether it is legitimate to lie for the sake of charity was a milestone, for in his disagreement with Benjamin Constant, Kant held that we are not even allowed to lie to a murderer asking us whether our friend he is pursuing is hiding in our house.[4] I wanted to explore the possibility that Kant's intransigence, projected backward, might be allied with Protestant-Puritan stances and opposed to moral casuistry on the Catholic side, which influenced medical thinking. In nonmedical literature, the two poles can be seen as represented in the Renaissance by Calvin's "anti-nicodemist" stance, as described in its context by Perez Zagorin (drawing in part on some work by Carlo Ginzburg) and the work of the canonists and moral casuists.[5] (2) In the Renaissance, the question whether falsehood was allowable in medicine had some status because Plato (who seemed to hold that it was) and Aristotle appeared to divide on it. (3) In a number of ways, the Renaissance discussions relate to problems discussed in our time, e.g. the question of placebos, of *fiducia* (i.e. the role of trust or confidence), of "openness" to the patients, etc. (4) Finally, and perhaps most important, many questions discussed in relation to pretense in curing relate to problems of imaginative literature, for not only was there a belief in the period that "the most feigning" literary work was the most true, but some of the greatest works of literature of that time are (or can profitably be considered) stories of curing.

Conceptions of medical ethics (even early and particularly Renaissance ones, as we shall see) often involve more than just the relationship between physician and patient. Dietrich von Engelhardt's diagram of the "structure of medical ethics" (adapted and translated from the German)[6] is not only a useful reminder of the possible relationships, but will enable us to see which are privileged in Renaissance medical speculation:

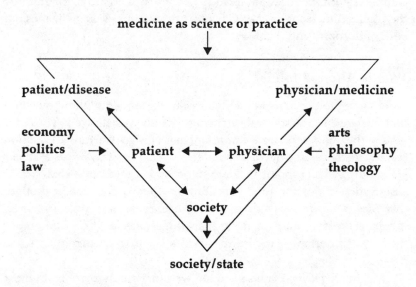

In the passages and recorded cases to be discussed (as in life), many of these relationships are present and expressed simultaneously. Since, for heuristic purposes, the following sections will isolate certain one-dimensional polarities (like physician:patient, physician: *adstantes*/society, physician:colleagues, etc.), the diagram is a useful reminder of the multiplicity of relationships. At the same time it is only a rough and preliminary roster, of course not specifically intended to express relationships operative in the Renaissance. Additions with which the skeletal roster will have to be fleshed out for that period should minimally include the *adstantes* (literally the persons "standing by" the patient's bed) as part of the society most immediately surrounding the sick, further licensing bodies of municipalities, the "midwife" acting as intermediary between physician and female patients with gynecological diseases (as we shall see in a later chapter), and the surgeon, by the academic physician considered of lower rank and sometimes presented as behaving unethically. That the spheres of philosophy/theology and politics/law appear linked and seemingly on opposing sides in this diagram is considerably more problematical, but should not preempt discussion of their relationship in later chapters, for that relationship was (and possibly still is) the most controverted. The advantage of this diagram over the one given by the physician Jeremias Cornarius in 1607 is that at least these complexes of influences are included, whereas Cornarius, diagraming the public dimension of the (Galenic) "rational physician," leaves out both philosophy and theology.[7]

Who Is Allowed to Lie?

Surely many physicians in the Renaissance assumed without question that pretense in the interest of curing was always allowed. Those for whom the matter became important enough to warrant discussion (as, for instance, Rodrigo a Castro [1546–1627] in his *Medicus-Politicus* [Hamburg, 1614]), point to Plato, who appears to have shared that assumption. Since for anyone writing on Renaissance medical ethics this *Medicus-Politicus* (written by a Portuguese Jew who practiced medicine in Hamburg for more than three decades) must be one of the most important texts, let me retrace Castro's argument in some detail.

In the *Republic*, Plato says that "we must surely prize truth most highly. For if we were right in what we were just saying, and falsehood is in very deed useless to gods, but to men useful as a remedy or form of medicine (*pharmakon*), it is obvious that such a thing must be assigned to physicians (*iatroi*), and laymen (*idiotai*) should have nothing to do with it. . . ."[8] Plato seems to assume that a falsehood as *pharmakon* is uncontroverted, since the point he is leading up to is that "the rulers then of the city may, if anybody, fitly lie on account of enemies or citizens for the benefit of state." In spite of the title of his book, Castro is not interested in this latter Platonic proposition (which has had an extraordinary fortune; see, for instance, Bacon's essay on dissimulation, which restricts everyone except kings and

princes to telling the truth), but in the medical implica.
pensation from truth. "Let's leave it to politics," he says.
point he agrees, although very cautiously, with the first hal.
he thinks is Plato's proposition quoted above, namely that dec
has a place in medicine, a view he finds confirmed in the Hippocr.
In epidemiis (or *De morb. vulg.*) and Galen's commentaries on that
work. Without quoting them, Castro in the margin refers to two passages from that work of the Hippocratic corpus: the cure of an earache by inserting into the ear wool dipped in oil and removing it in
such a manner as to trick the patient into believing that some other
substance has been removed (and immediately throwing it into the
fire, presumably destroying the evidence)—in this context the Hippocratic word is *apate* (deception, deceit, lie); and a passage exhorting
physicians to "gratify" the wishes of the patient, a mode much commended by Galen in his commentary.[10] Castro apparently summarizes these passages by saying that Hippocrates "in *Epidemiis* seems to
recommend deception rather frequently, and Galen in his commentary adds that sometimes one has to resort to falsehoods."[11] For whatever reason, Castro is more than a little imprecise here: Galen had
questioned the deception advocated in the Hippocratic earache story
to the point of surmising that the passage was spurious.

The sick, Castro says (following traditional thinking), are by
nature suspicious and fearful, not only intently listening to each word
of the physician, but in their concern also screening the physician's
face for clues. Therefore the prudent physician (*medicus prudens*) will
try to cover or conceal by simulation (*simulatione tegere*) whatever
might add to the patients' fears or perturb their mind. Since (as he
says with Celsus) one needs to make the sick secure, so that they suffer only physically and not mentally, it is best to withhold from them
what might upset them. How to deal with a fearful (*timidus*) patient
had very much been the concern of the ancient physicians. In his commentary on the Hippocratic passage urging that the physician gratify
the patients' wishes (cited above), Galen had said that only patients
who were prudent and not "fearful" would be given an actual prognosis without "subtracting" and "dissimulating" anything. On Castro's choice of words, it should be noted, that his use of *simulatione
tegere* seems to indicate that he is not abiding by the somewhat techni-
cal distinction some of his contemporaries made between *simulatio*
(pretending the presence of something that is not there) and *dissimulatio* (pretending that something that is present is not there).[12]

Celsus's phrase about placating or appeasing the patients' minds so as to concentrate on the cure of the body may seem innocent and uncontroversial enough—after all, even the papal mandate obliging a Catholic physician to urge his patients to confession before undertaking any cure was not understood as a means to secure their passage to a happy afterlife, but to remove whatever interfered with recovery, since sin could be a cause of sickness.[13] However, as we will see later, in other contexts than in Protestant Hamburg (where Castro published all his books), he might have been on thin ice with the recommendation to withhold matters from the notice of the sick in order not to upset their minds. Castro then sharpens his proposition by referring to Damascenus' aphorisms that one should always promise the patient health even when one has given up hope.

Thus it would seem that Castro believes that patients are "different," so different in fact that ordinary rules of communication are suspended. Although he will eventually subscribe to that view, he first tries to justify, in a detour that will call for comment in a later chapter, the constant expression of confidence (in recovery) as *simulatio*: "For simulation, in which truth is withheld by silence or is wrapped as by a veil, is one thing; it is another thing to express as true something that is false. The former is not only without guilt, but in its time and place is considered laudable and virtuous."[14] As example of such licit *simulatio* he gives David's ruse of changing his behavior and feigning madness in order to escape from Achish, the king of Gath, when he feared for his life (1 Sam. 21:13).

Perhaps Castro realized that by referring to the promising of health in spite of better knowledge as "simulation" he was inordinately stretching the meaning of that word, for at this point he takes another step: he says that according to "most" (*plerique*), the physician must not only simulate and pretend (*fingere*), but even use lies in order that the patient recover by art. According to him, this is what Galen did when, under the pretense of giving a woman whey, he had her drink scammony.[15] "We" do something similar still, Castro tells us, when we give children or dejected patients pomegranate juice instead of wine or quite generally conceal unpleasant ingredients in other potions or hide from them the death of relatives or the loss of goods and instead substitute what is cheerful for what is sad, or when we pretend (*fingere*) to recalcitrant patients that their ills are more serious than they really are to bring them to a more reasonable style of life and to have them accept medical assistance: "So a collapsed

uterus [prolapse?] is often brought back to its proper plac
strative showing of the hot cauterizing iron, and in extreme .
not seem improper to speak other than one really feels so that t.
one is not driven to despair."[16] Then he draws once more on Gan
commentary on Hippocrates by citing Galen's view that the sick
should be made to obey by amplifying their maladies (*maiores fin-
genda vitia*) and, where the truth does not do the job, even by threatening, scaring, and evocation of danger.

But as Castro dramatizes the controversy, "Aristotle fights for
the other side" (p. 143), for in his *Nicomachean Ethics*, Aristotle praises
truthfulness in itself, even when nothing depends on it (bk. 4, chap.
7), and considers contemptible any lying whatsoever. In addition,
Castro quotes Pythagoras (from Aelianus' *Variae historiae libri XIV*) as
having said that humans had received these outstanding gifts from
God: to tell the truth and do good to others. Lying, however, is an
evil, and therefore nothing good can come from it. It is contrary to the
order of God and of nature (*ordo Dei et naturae*), for since words are
given to humankind as signs of what is in the mind, it is against
nature that someone express by them what is not there or even contrary to what is there. Castro also uses Paul's phrase (Rom. 3:8),
which is a commonplace of Renaissance moral speculation (certainly
also of the moral casuistry of the Jesuits): *Non sunt facienda mala ut eveniant bona* (evil is not to be done that good may come out of it, or the
end does not justify the means).[17]

But then Castro takes an important turn. Exploring the other
side of the coin, he gives three reasons why certain types of untruth-
fulness should be allowed. First, he says that it is not only *not* blame-
worthy in a certain place and at a certain time to be silent about the
truth, but it is even laudable. Second, there is a vast difference
between a harmful lie and an "officious" lie (*mendacium nocivum et
mendacium officiosum*). While the former is always to be avoided and
condemned, the second produces in the listener a meaning that,
though false, is most useful, for one always needs to consider both
intent and meaning: not just what someone did, but why and for
what purpose. For that reason, he reports, lying has been compared to
hellebore: taken without necessity and without utmost discrimination, it is deadly; but in the circumstance of a deadly disease, it is salu-
tary. According to Castro, lies should similarly be used "like a
medication or a condiment" (*uti medicamentum et condimentum*), i.e.
one should never lie, if I understand his Latin correctly, "without

great usefulness for one's neighbor" (*sine maxima proximi utilitate*). Third, Castro finds additional support in the notion of *dolus* (ruse, cleverness), which according to traditional speculation can be good or bad, the "good" ruse being the one justified against an enemy or a robber.

In his *Quaestiones medico-legales* (Rome, 1634), the Roman Catholic physician and very subtle medical ethicist Zacchia (1584–1659), who is interested in defining the culpable *dolus malus* of the physician, will avoid Castro's terminological awkwardness about two types of *mendacium* and make do with the conventional legal term *dolus* (lib. 6, tit. 1, quaestiones 1–2). For Castro has to claim that Aristotle and Pythagoras had in mind only "useless" or "harmful" lies. From then on, of course, Castro has clear sailing: "Let the assertion be firm that the physician is allowed to pretend (*fingere*) anything for the sake of a person's health, to dissemble (*dissimulare*) and also to promise what may strengthen the patient's spirit" (p. 144). He even adduces the examples, entirely topical in this context, of Jacob pretending to be Esau (Gen. 27:19) and of the midwives lying to Pharaoh to save the children (Ex. 1:17–20), suggesting (rather than arguing in any detail) that they are instances of justified deception, before breaking off and admitting, as was customary on all sides of the religious spectrum: "But these are examples of a contemplation more divine and high and of a more secret sense."[18]

Thus, although Castro at first teases out a difference of opinion between Plato and Aristotle, he shows ultimately that the two can be reconciled: Aristotle did not have in mind these justified ruses. And Plato's view of the lying *pharmakon*, taken by him as axiomatic to Plato's thought, is not seen as enough of a foundation: the ancient legal thinking about the *dolus ad bonum* is an attempt to find the broadest possible basis.

Castro directly expresses notions that many physicians only imply. We will encounter again the notion of *dolus* in Alfonso Ponce de Santacruz' (fl. 1600) idea of the *medicus fingens* as clever strategist: for here the clever outmaneuvering of the enemy (analogous to the disease) is assumed as axiomatically justified, and I mentioned that Zacchia manages to arrive at commonsensical conclusions similar to Castro's without the awkwardness of a dichotomized lie (*mendacium*).

But the common-sense nature of these solutions can easily be overstressed. Before I get into details of medical choices and ethical comment (under three rough headings: the need to deceive the medical colleague, the patient, and the world around the patient), I would like to point to Giovanni Battista Cortesi's (1554–1636) reading of the passage from the *Republic* that Castro, and probably most readers, saw as endorsing the deceitful use of medication to bring about a cure. It will be recalled that after saying that falsehood was useless to the gods and useful to men only as a medication, Plato had restricted the use of this medication to the physician and wanted it kept out of the hands of private men (*idiotai*). He had further said that rulers, if anybody, may lie for the benefit of the state; but for private or lay men to lie was as nonsensical as for patients to conceal something from their physician or for a sailor to deceive his pilot. In his reinterpretation of the passage, Cortesi dichotomizes "physicians" thus:[19]

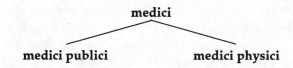

The point of the division is to say that Plato is talking about *medici publici* and not at all about physicians in the strict sense. The latter, according to Cortesi, have no dispensation from truthfulness. He claimed to base his reading on Ficino (1433–1499), the most celebrated expositor of Plato, and indeed, in summarizing the *argumentum* of the dialogue, Ficino had clarified what we might call the class- or power-determined nature of Plato's view, in which lying is taken as a calamity of society when *privati* lie to one another, but especially when they lie to their magistrates (which, following Plato, he likened to patients lying to their doctor or sailors to their pilot)—while pilots were allowed to lie for the public good.[20] But Ficino, to my knowledge, had not commented on or explained away the notion of falsehood as a "pharmakon," the crucial medical term Plato used to introduce the distinction between the use of lying by those in power (*medici publici*, physicians only in a manner of speaking) and by those ruled by power.

The reinterpretation by Cortesi, who rose from barber to barber-surgeon to physician and professor of medicine, is not an act of mere academic rereading of an ancient passage but an apology for his profession: an act of enhancing the reputation of doctors and at the same time of castigating a colleague who, by his deceitful practice, has caused the profession some disrepute. Like many of the cases I will discuss, this one exemplifies various relations operative in the triangle given above, of which I privilege at this point the physician's relationship to colleagues.

The Physician and His Colleagues

Cortesi tells the case of a doctor who, called to the bed of a female patient seriously ill, proclaimed that the other physicians consulted had entirely misdiagnosed her illness and had failed to treat it properly. This doctor further predicted, not only to the noble lady's relatives but to all the nobility at court, that with his treatment she would soon recover. Her husband and family were overjoyed by this prognosis, and letters were sent to distant relatives assuring them that the patient was safe since a famous physician had said so. For some time the physician was praised to the sky, while the other doctors were held in low esteem. But after a brief period of remission, the patient died. "In order to vindicate himself, the *anomalus* wrote in his little book that on the authority of Plato's *Republic*, public physicians (*publici medici*) were allowed to lie" (p. 763). It is to counter such flagrant malpractice and flippant justification that Cortesi engages in the hermeneutic act by which he will show that the *medici publici* Plato meant were not clinical physicians but political leaders.

Relationships among physicians naturally become a topic in the collections of *consultationes* that have come down to us and in the works specifically outlining the theory and practice of consulting colleagues, e.g. Giovanni Argenterio (1513–1572). *De consultationibus medicis sive (ut vulgus vocat) de collegiandi ratione liber* (Florence, 1551). Here deceit is addressed in Argenterio's complaint that some colleagues appear to try to impress others by talking about nothing but medical authorities (p. 123) rather than persuading by reason and experience—Argenterio often was very critical of Galen and, as a consequence, particularly sensitive to the practice of quoting him by a "simulated erudition" (*simulata eruditio*, p. 13). Castro observes from the opposite perspective (that of the "rational" physician) that some people who pass for physicians know no learned language nor any *ethica philosophia*, but have learned a few morsels by heart (p. 72).

By its tactics of composition, much of Renaissance medical writing is aimed at the "errors" of other physicians, and persons persist-

ing in error are considered morally culpable. Thus Giovanni Filippo
Ingrassias (1510–1580) writes to correct medical *errors*, and his *Iatrapologia* (c. 1550) is by its subtitle programmatically directed against "barbaric" physicians: *Liber quo multa adversus barbaros medicos, collegiique
modus ostenditur.* Furthermore, Castro explains the purpose of his *Medicus-Politicus*, which was dedicated to the Hamburg senate, through a
similarly descriptive title as "a treatise . . . expressing not only the habits and virtues of good physicians but also exposing the deceptions
and impostures of the bad ones."[21] To some extent, to call the incapable colleagues pretenders or actors is an old topos, inherited from
ancient medicine. Pietro Castelli (1590–1661), very much a defender of
Hippocrates, adduces and rephrases the Hippocratic passage already
referred to when he says that "such [bad] physicians are very similar
to actors on the tragic stage. For they have the look, behavior, and the
mask of those they represent, but they are not the very ones. Thus
many are physicians by reputation and in name, but few are in
reality."[22]

But the uses to which these allegations are put are not necessarily commonplace. The question who can or should be consulted naturally has to do with defining bona fide colleagues as different from
"fakes." From the point of view of "rational" physicians, the "empirical" and "chemical" doctors and healers are often seen as "vultures"
(*vulturii*), as Meibom (1590–1655) puts it, who surround both the
credulous rich lords and the inexperienced common people.[23] These
shameful contrivers (*pravi artifices*) give medicine a bad name
(Castro, p. 72). Like the surgeon Paré and the physician Joubert
before him, and many other physicians addressing the authorities of
their city, Castro would like certain of his "colleagues" to be excluded
from practice. Characteristically, it had been in a chapter entitled "De
certains imposteurs," chock full of examples of malpractice, that Paré
had addressed himself to the *magistrats*.[24] Castro's *Medicus-Politicus* is
political in the modern sense in that the author is implicitly urging
the Hamburg patricians to be more discriminating about whom they
allow to practice.

Although not very general, there is a distinct thread in Renaissance medical writing warning patients and colleagues to be critical
rather than credulous of medical opinion. In *The Key to Unknowne
Knowledge* (a medical compendium purporting to consist of Hippocrates' *De natura humana* with Jean de Bourges' annotations, an interesting but "supposititious" work), the author encourages the women

he addresses to observe their bodies carefully and not to trust the word of the physician, who may not recognize a pregnancy. Their trust in physicians who, to "put themselves into credit," pretend certainty where there is none, may endanger their offspring:

> ... which seemeth a matter of conscience, and I would not set it downe, if I had not seene it proved, and by the helpe of God remedied, that such mischiefe might not happen. Wherefore you women wheresoever you bee, when you perceave anie signe of greatnesse or conceaving with child, I pray you hazard it not, for although by the water some apparent signes may bee, it is impossible that the Physician whatsoever hee be, can assure thee, by meanes of thy water onelie.[25]

While critiques of uroscopy in the sixteenth century are frequent—one of the few changes in actual diagnostic practice in the period is the degradation of uroscopy—this text is somewhat unusual in being addressed to the patients rather than the scholarly community. In fact, the author takes a dim view of his colleagues, whom he calls not only ignorant but arrogant, and encourages the patients (possibly still primarily women) to get a second opinion, compare consultations, and have physicians justify their diagnoses:

> Wherefore if thou chaunce to call them unto consultation, I counsell thee to cause them to speake by order: and if there happen anie contrarietie among them (which is often done, more for the glorie of the world, then [sic] for the health of the partie) then it is expedient for thee to cause them to yeeld a reason for their sayings, to the end the wise and expert Physician may be knowne from the asse and audacious foole. (sig. K)

This is strong language, and one wonders whether for this reason the author of the book did not clearly identify himself.

Since there had been a string of papal pronouncements against Jewish providers of medical care (including pharmacists), the physician Codronchi's important *De Christiana ac tuta medendi ratione* (1591), a book close to the views and temperaments of Catholic moral casuists (as we will see later), includes an entire chapter on restrictions Christian physicians and patients should observe in consulting Jewish doctors. It was a mortal sin for the Christian physician to consult, or for the Christian patient to call, a Jewish doctor. But Codronchi makes an important and characteristically casuistic exculpating exception "when necessity obliges one to call them, namely where there aren't any Christian physicians or ones appropriately equipped for curing a particular disease."[26] One of the justifications for excluding Jews was the belief, transmitted through folk motifs from medieval literature, that they preyed on Christians by ruses and deceit (Codronchi, p. 112).

Although warnings against deceitful chemical and empirical healers were commonplace in the writings of the academic or "rational" physicians, opinions as to who could be "consulted" differed widely. According to Ranchin (1565–1641), who was particularly astute in questions of medical ethics and, like Meibom, had written a commentary on the Hippocratic oath, even *empyrici*, *operatores* (barber surgeons?), and midwives could and should be consulted in extreme cases.[27] Women are particularly to be heard "when women out of modesty reject the services of the surgeons" (p. 707). Similarly, although Laurent Joubert (1529–1582) spends much time documenting malpractice by women (caused by arrogance, deceit, or ignorance), he is willing to cede the area of childbirth to the women (whom he calls *matrones* and *levandières*) for reasons of modesty—as long as they will work under the supervision of the approved physician:

> However, we cede to them the part of surgery relating to childbirth; for it is more proper (*honeste*) that that particular work involving the pudenda (*ez parties honteuses*) be done from woman to woman....[28]

In a similar vein, it was apparently no contradiction for Johannes Molanus (1533–1585) to include a female saint and healer *medicinae perita* in his ecclesiastical calendar of physicians and at the same time (and on the same page) to object to allowing women to study medicine.[29]

To illustrate some of these issues (and supply at the same time an example of studied pretense and apparently even in Renaissance terms justified deception of medical colleagues), I will quote a story often cited in the Renaissance and originating with the second century writer Hyginus. Just as with the classical passages I cited earlier, we must keep in mind that classical learning in this period is not merely an antiquarian matter but often supplies the signposts of orientation for the present. The story is about a young woman of Athens who, in order to circumvent a supposedly Athenian law forbidding slaves and women to exercise the art of surgery, cuts her hair, puts on male clothes, and enters the service of a physician. Although modern translations are available, I quote Hyginus's account from Thomas Heywood's *Gynaikeion* (1624), starting from the point at which she has learned the art of medicine from her male mentor:

> By her industrie and studie having attained to the deapth of his skill and the height of her own desires, upon a time hearing where a noble ladie was in child-birth, in the middest of her painfull throwes, she offered her selfe to her helpe, whom the modest Ladie (mistaking her Sex) would by no persuasion suffer to come neere her, till she was forced to strip her selfe before the women, and to give evident signes of her woman-hood. After which she had access to many, prooving so fortunate, that she grew verie famous. In so much that being envied by the colledge of Phisitians, she was complained on to the Areopagitae, or the nobilitie of the Senat: such in whose power it was to censure and determine of all causes and controversies. *Agnodice* thus convented, they pleaded against her youth and boldnesse, accursing her rather a corrupter of their chastities, than any way a curer of their infirmities: blaming the matrons, as counterfeiting weaknesse, onely of purpose to have the companie and familiaritie of a loose and intemperate yong man. They prest their accusations so far, that the Iudges were readie to procede to sentence against her; when she opening her brest before the Senat, gave manifest testimonie that she was no other than a woman: at this the Phisitians the more incenst made the fact the more henious, in regard that being a woman, she durst enter into the search of that knowledge, of which their Sex by the law was not capable. The cause being once more readie to goe against her, the noble matrons of the cittie assembled before the Senat, and plainely told them, they were rather enemies than husbands, who went about to punish her, that of all their Sex had beene most studious for their generall health and safetie. Their importancie so farre prevailed, after the circumstances were truely considered, that the first decree was quite abrogated, and free libertie granted to women to imploy themselves in those necessary offices, without the presence of men. So that

Athens was the first cittie of Greece, that freely admitted of Midwives by the meanes of this damosell *Agnodice* (p. 204).

The story would merit analysis on a number of levels: the historical and mythical levels, both of which were addressed to some extent by Campbell Bonner, who claimed that the statement that the
ancients had no midwives was absurd and was convinced that "wise
women" treated minor ailments with impunity. He considered the
story therefore a novella of popular origin, sharing, for instance, with
the Christian legend of St. Eugenia the elements of cross-dressing and
"exposure as apotropaeic gesture."[30] A different level of interest entirely, and much closer to my concerns, would be in the reception of
the Hagnodice story in the Renaissance. For it seems to have been
quite well known and taken for fact, as appears from Girolamo Bardi's (1600–1667) inclusion of Hagnodice among famous female physicians. (Bardi was a priest turned physician, and in a later chapter I
will argue that his *Medicus politico Catholicus* was written in response
to Castro's *Medicus-Politicus*.)[31] Heywood emphasizes the envy and
even malice of her male colleagues and renders with apparent satisfaction the successful class or sisterhood action of the Athenian
women. It is to be doubted that Bonner would have arrived at his
ideas on the apotropaeic and aischrological core of the story on the basis of the English version, for Heywood does not have Hagnodice lift
her tunic twice, but has her demonstrate her sex considerably more
modestly.[32]

Why would there have been such sympathy for Hagnodice's
deception of her medical colleagues in an age that by all accounts was
authoritarian and rarely rewarded the circumventer of laws and professional rules? The story could be read and was read as an account of
how midwives, not female physicians, came to be allowed, an
account, in other words, of how the status quo had been achieved.
Thus it was not necessarily an anecdote presenting a revolutionary
model, but it recorded clearly that many women prefer and may need
to receive medical attention from women, a point that is only beginning to be recognized fully in our age. However, it has to be said that
with his view that women are capable of pursuing all branches of
knowledge, Bardi is at the radical end of this spectrum.

The anecdote about the cross-dressing Hagnodice presented in
traditional language as female modesty the desire of women to be
treated by women but not the extreme reaction of the saint (that later

ages might find quaint and Protestant England, objectionable), as in the instance of St. Agatha who, unwilling to show her body, refused the help of physicians and of physic.[33] Given the records we have, this need is usually represented (as in the passage I cited from Joubert) as male willingness to allow women to deal with what is considered improper or unclean. (We will discuss this subject in more detail in a later chapter.) The story of Hagnodice is unusual in that with the women assembling in the Areopagus and accusing their husbands of trying to undo the very woman who, by circumventing existing laws, has healed them, it expresses the gynecological area not negatively but from the female perspective as an area requiring female medical attention and the confidence of the female patient. Equally notable is the fact that with all her cunning, Hagnodice manages to resolve her dilemma by keeping the physician–patient relationship free from pretense or falsehood. She deceives only her "colleagues."

Physician and Patient

I earlier mentioned Alfonso Ponce de Santacruz's notion of the *medicus fingens*. Santacruz (fl. 1600) likens the physician to the "dexterous military leader trying to overcome some hostile fortress" (*strenuus militiae dux arcem aliquam oppugnaturus*), and pursues the analogy at considerable length.[34] We also recall that in warfare deception is traditionally and almost axiomatically allowed, i.e. the *dolus* is most likely *dolus ad bonum*. In the interest of health, says Julius Alexandrinus (or Alessandrini, 1506–1590), "let us lie healthily . . . as it was never shameful for leaders of armies or princes of states to lie in the interest of their armies and states."[35]

 Although in this model not the patient but the disease is the enemy, the entire concept results in some ingenious inventions, and physicians act like stage managers, cleverly changing the behavior of the patients by "trickery" in the interest of a desired cure. Such therapy is indicated only in particular pathological conditions, namely in what was called melancholy, specifically a kind of melancholy conceived as *laesa imaginatio*. In this condition the hurt or injured imagination is supposed to be healed by the imagination itself. Modern readers are perhaps most familiar with this therapy "by deceit" through the works of Cervantes (both *Don Quixote* and "El Licenciado Vidriera" of the *Novelas exemplares* are closely related to this medical

theory and practice).[36] I may begin by relating some particulars of
this therapy before progressing to the critical issues it raised for
Renaissance physicians. Their critiques will perhaps seem so arcane
that they would never occur to a modern psychiatrist, but for that
very reason (since they bespeak a different frame of reference) they
are instructive to the modern historian.

Some of the oldest reported cases of melancholics are the ones of
persons thinking their body a receptacle of brittle substance (*vas,
figulum*) and not allowing anyone near them, of people thinking themselves birds and moving their arms like wings, and of people imagining that they are laboring with other animals within their bodies,
usually snakes or frogs. Galen's brief catalogue in *De locis affectis* (bk.
3, chap. 10, Kühn ed., vol. 8, pp. 190–90) includes the man imagining
his body is brittle (a breakable vessel or shell) and therefore avoiding
human contact, the bird man, and the person thinking that he is Atlas
holding up the world, but Galen does not mention whether or how
these patients were cured (except that the context might be read to
suggest venisection and purgation). Probably the case from the
Hippocratic corpus of curing an earache by the ruse of pretending to
remove some peccant substance from the ear belongs to this tradition,
as the Renaissance commentator in the edition adduced earlier surmised. In other words, this was not a case of curing an earache, but a
therapy for someone imagining one. Cases like these are fleshed out
with detail in the Renaissance and are collected in such works as Marcello Donati's *De medica historia mirabili* (1586) and Ercole Sassonia's
(or Saxonia, 1551–1607) *De melancholia*, c. 8 (1620). These titles are
merely illustrative; such cases are almost invariably part of the section
"De *melancholia*" of Renaissance books on medicine, and it would
therefore be tedious to list them. Not all the works giving examples of
melancholy characterized as *laesa imaginatio*, however, report a therapy; since my subject is the physician's ruse or deception in treating
the patient, I am going to concentrate on only the most ingenious ther-
apeutic procedures I have found reported in the period.

Perhaps the palm should go to Zacuto's (1575–1642) *observatio*
entitled *Melancholicus artificio curatus* (A melancholic cured by an
artifice). Zacuto tells the case of a young Portuguese of dark complex-
ion, sad, and of a meditative bent, who suddenly without any warning, conceived the melancholic fantasy (*melancholiam imaginationem*)
that his sins would never be forgiven by God. He persisted in this
agony for eight months, during which he suffered dangerous weight

loss. Women practicing various kinds of wonderful cures and magic medicine could not help him. When at the desperation point physicians were consulted, he preached to them day and night about God being the only hinge of his salvation, without whom he was sure he would end up with the devil, to whom he talked every day. The physicians agreed on a therapy by purgation, bloodletting by application of leeches and other means "that use to be prescribed for insomnia, weight loss and dejection." But nothing helped, and the patient rejected all wholesome counsel from friends and all sport that was meant to distract him. "But when we had seen that all of this had been thoughtfully done, yet in vain, we used another artful stratagem." After some tiles of the roof had first been carefully loosened, an ostensible angel (*angelus arteficialis*) appeared to the patient in the dead of the night, dressed in white, carrying in his right hand a sword and in his left a burning torch. When he called the patient's name three times, the melancholic rose from his bed and, prostrate on the ground, venerated the angel, who proceeded to reveal to him that by the grace of the Almighty all his sins were forgiven. Then the visitor extinguished his torch and disappeared. According to Zacuto, the ruse worked: the young man immediately reported his vision to his relatives, then to his doctors, who congratulated him and called him justified (*iustum*). He also started to eat and entirely recovered. "Therefore, if melancholics cannot be cured by art [of medicine], then by industry and we need to use deception by which, as experience teaches us, they can be healed."[37]

No less ingenious and more often rehearsed in the medical literature of the period is the cure of a melancholic who believed not that he was dying but that he was already dead, and therefore hid in a cellar, refusing any nourishment. At a desperate hour of his decline, a friend of his had a table close by set with the most appetizing food and drink and started to eat and drink within hearing of his friend, whom he invited to join him. When the melancholic refused again by saying that he was dead, the friend retorted that so was he, but that the dead also ate. By this reasoning, the melancholic was persuaded to join him and accept life-preserving nourishment.[38]

Renaissance medical works that explain the cure of the imagination by the imagination invariably refer to persons who are laboring under the conviction that they are harboring a frog, snake, or bird in some part of their body being cured by the physician or his assistant surreptitiously slipping such an animal into a bowl for display while they are being purged. That the theory of such therapy by trickery, and perhaps even the practice, was indeed standard is borne out by the report (1609) by the Swiss physician Felix Platter, whose "melancholic" patient exclaimed while being purged: "You can't do that to me!" Alerted by his own medical studies on the subject, this patient had caught sight of an assistant readying a live frog for show.[39]

Quite high on my scale of ingenuity (second only because of its traditional core) is the case represented by Alfonso de Santacruz (who, as I mentioned, compares the physician to a military strategist) as coming from a medical teacher of his at Paris, namely the cure of a melancholic who thought his body was of glass (*vas vitreum*). The "most prudent physician (*prudentissimus medicus*), who knew that the patient was incessantly worried that his limbs might be shattered, cunningly suggested to him that he sleep on straw. When [the patient] did, the physician found a pretext to visit him in his room, set a match to the straw and quickly left the room, locking the door. Desperately rapping at the door, the patient finally yelled: 'Open up, friends, I beseech you. . . . For I am not of glass any more but think myself the most miserable of humans particularly if you leave me to this fire to take my life.' For his fear that the flames would consume him was so intense that it caused his false imagination to vanish."[40] This radical therapy can profitably be compared with another invention for which Abraham Zacuto claims credit. When asked to treat a melancholic imagining himself always to be cold and freezing to death (he had already three times tried to jump into a fire), he "devised the following remedy" (*hoc sum machinatus auxilium*): he had him clothed in sheepskin that had been soaked in *aqua vitae*. After a match was set to him, the patient burned like a torch for half a hour while jumping about enjoying the heat, until he shouted he was sane and too warm. "And thus, with that imagination removed, he was restored to health within a few days."[41]

Other than the scale of ingenuity, a criterion of questionable objectivity and no explanatory power, the last two examples suggest a grouping of such psychiatric cases on another scale (which I have explored in different contexts), namely the scale from gentleness at one end (in cases where the patient is somehow cured by the example of gentle persuasion of a *socius* or *amicus* who joins him) to fear and even terror on the other (where the intensity of one element of the imagination is thought to cancel another).

At best, however, such scales are occasionally implied by the authors citing these cases—they are hardly ever made explicit. Therefore, it may be instructive to glance at the questions Thomas Fienus (or Feyens [1567–1631], whose *De viribus imaginationis* was invariably praised for its acumen) distills from these and similar medical cases. As Fienus surveys the kind of cases we have discussed (i.e. patients healed by trickery of their conviction that they have swallowed frogs or snakes), he insists that these are special cases of melancholic imagination in which the patients are healed by virtue of their firm confidence and intense (sometimes he says "high") imagination. Fienus's concerns emerge most clearly in his rejection of the sixteenth-century physician Thomás da Veiga's analysis of a seemingly similar case: here a patient in a delirium had frequently and obstinately asked his physicians to allow him to dip into "that pool" (*illud stagnum*)—he was pointing down to the dry pavement where he imagined water— saying that only then would he recover. The moment they granted him his wish, he threw himself down onto the pavement, where, after tumbling about for some time, he said with joy: "Now it's up to my knees." When he thought the water reached to his throat, he said he was healthy and, according to the source, had indeed been healed.[42]

Fienus insists that it would be a mistake to assume that the patient was healed by the imagination, because the imagination cannot heal. To assume otherwise would mean not to take seriously the distinction between body and soul and thus, if I read him correctly, to lapse into some form of heresy. For to admit that the imagination actually heals the body would obliterate that distinction and ultimately— this emerges from the nature of his examples and the persistence with which he drives home the point—admit magic. Thus the recovery of the imagined swimmer was *casuale* or, as he puts it elsewhere (using scholastic vocabulary), *per accidens*, but not *causale*. We simply do not know why the man recovered, Fienus explains; possibly the chill of the pavement cured his fever (pp. 199–200), for bodily melancholy, which only is truly a disease, cannot be healed by devices (*inventa*, p. 200). Although the distinction may seem arcane to some modern readers and even a disappointment to those who have come to appreciate the psychosomatic nexus in much humoral physiology, the point was crucial to "rational" physicians (thinking in an Aristotelian tradition) like Laurentius (Du Laurens, ca. 1550–1609) and Fienus, setting them and many of their colleagues off from others writing in the more "magical" tradition of Marsilio Ficino and Cornelius Agrippa. While, as Nancy Siraisi has shown, versions of this issue were discussed in medieval Italy in the circle around Taddeo Alderotti (and to some extent were a standard topic of theoretical medicine), the competition of Paracelsian and alchemical medicine and its customary Protestant inclination may have given the problem a particular ideological urgency in the early seventeenth century.[43]

This philosophical problem, whose practical implications I cannot pursue any further, bears on a topic that must be addressed in my context, namely in what sense the relationship between patient and physician was conceived as fiduciary in a general and not necessarily legal sense. Renaissance medical writers indeed often discuss *fiducia* as an important concept in the physician-patient relationship, but with the exception of commentaries on the "Hippocratic oath," which do of course mention what the physician may and may not do to the patient's dependents and property, they are almost exclusively concerned with insisting that the patient's confidence contributes importantly to the cure. Michael Boudewyns (1606–1681), who at the end of the period summarizes (in this case somewhat uncritically) earlier discussions, writes about the persuasive power of autosuggestion and cites Avicenna's (ca. 979–1034) dictum: *Illum medicum curare, cui plurimum confidunt* (The physician in whom there is most trust works cures). Similarly, in his chapter 15, "De fiducia in medicum et quaedam cautela," Galeotto Marzio (1450–1497) rehearses traditional pronouncements on this subject (by Hippocrates, Galen, Rhasis, and others), and it is tempting to dismiss many such discussions as medical commonplace.[44] But Fienus's discussions of the powers of the imagination and the particular and practical advice that is sometimes derived from notions of *fiducia* persuade me that such dismissal would be a mistake.

Fienus offers perhaps the most extensive collection of pronouncements and examples of what wonders the patient's belief or confidence can work in the process of healing. They include Pomponazzi's (1462–1525) "daring" pronouncement that the cures by saints' bones could also have been effected by the bones of dogs (p. 192)—a view that may have been shared by Chaucer's Pardoner in the *Canterbury Tales*—and the pronouncement Fienus attributes to Albertus Magnus (1193–1280), namely that the sick can cure themselves by confidence in their physician as much as the physicians cure by medications (p. 191). But for reasons I have touched on, Fienus's radical Aristotelianism in this sense makes him play the role of an early *Aufklärer*, or precursor of the Enlightenment, debunking magic and the use of amulets and incantations—Fienus rejects these claims as overblown: the imagination by itself cannot cure; Pomponazzi spoke "impiously" (for good reason his book is indexed by the Holy See, Fienus says), and Albertus Magnus sinned by attributing too much power to the imagination (p. 198). At present, I find it difficult to determine whether many physicians shared Fienus's skepticism, although he undoubtedly had a high reputation (Robert Burton [1577–1640], for instance, invariably refers to him with high praise). Certainly the important writer François Ranchin (1565–1641), in a similar context, also goes on the attack against Avicenna, Paracelsus, and the Cabalists. It may be significant that from 1593 Fienus taught medicine at Louvain, which would have been at that time at the center of the rise of neo-scholasticism in the wake of the Council of Trent.[45]

Those who emphasize the role of the imagination and the function of *fiducia* in therapy, however, tend to let this notion control their idea of the doctor's entire procedure at the sickbed: his appearance, demonstrated frame of mind, and accommodation to the patient's habits in the interest of a *captatio benevolentiae* (as is pointed out by Julius Alexandrinus [1506–1590], author of what may be one of the first books of medical ethics).[46] In the margin (p. 334), Alexandrinus summarizes his argument concisely as, "One is allowed to lie for the health of the patient" (*Licere mentiri pro salute laborantis*), and, "The sick person's respect is to be won" (*Benevolentia aegri captanda*).

From the observation that the sick are healed primarily by *fiducia* Galeotto Marzio ultimately derives even the conclusion that it is "most useful for the common and ignorant that one speak to them in Punic or Greek or some other language they do not understand."[47] For, as this physician explains, it happened to him in Bohemia, Germany, Hungary, and Spain that, asked by patients what medication he was preparing for them, when he answered using Punic or some other language he spoke, the patients recovered. Extreme as Marzio's reasoning may be, there seems to have been a consensus in the Renaissance that, as Leonardo Botallo (1530–1587) puts it in his book on the duties of physician and patient, "it is . . . proper that the physician not reveal the composition of medications to the sick and their helpers."[48] While Botallo's interest may be primarily to guard professional secrets, their safeguard could easily be justified by the larger principle of strengthening the patients' *fiducia*.

If the operation of *fiducia* between doctor and patient in Renaissance medical ethics is usually conceived as the patient's trust in the physician's ability, there is one important exception where many accounts focus on the physician's duty to the patient (although the Renaissance texts I have seen do not treat this problem literally under the word *fiducia*): it is the discussion of whether the physician must tell the terminally ill the truth about their condition. The full impact of this problem can only be grasped against the background of two emphases emerging specifically from medicine in the context of Christianity: a new sense of medical obligation to the terminally or incurably ill (as opposed to injunctions in Greek medicine warning the physician against treating patients he cannot cure) and a sense of responsibility (insisted on by Roman Catholic authors, in accordance with papal mandate) for encouraging a Christian to make use of the last rites and sacraments before dying.[49]

My remarks are of course intended to differentiate Christian medicine from that of the Greeks, not from Hebrew or even Muslim traditions, in which the emphasis on charity may be equally strong. In fact, Immanuel Jakobovits has claimed that in Judaism the principle of avoiding avoidable pain is so strong that it overrides other concerns:

> A medical illustration of this principle occurs in the story of the Syrian King Ben Hadad, whose messenger Hazael, sent to inquire from the Prophet Elisha whether the king would survive his sickness, was told: "Go say unto him 'You shall surely recover;' howbeit the Lord has shown me that he shall surely die" (2 Kings 8:10). Jewish ethics in some respects regards peace as an even greater virtue than truth; hence it rates the patient's peace of mind higher than the doctor's truthfulness if this might undermine the patient's hope or mental tranquility.[50]

Although Jakobovits's interpretation of Elisha's motives is debatable (as I will show further on), the passage can serve as a first illustration of the kind of dilemmas physicians face, balancing a multiplicity of interests: from the deontological principle to be truthful to a variety of other principles and interests.

If we look at how Codronchi, in the Renaissance often cited on medical ethics, conceptualizes the Christian physician's dilemma, we see that it would be a mistake to think of his plight as a conflict between charity and Church requirements or between appeasing the patient versus appeasing the Church, for these interests are interpreted to be the same. To make someone aware of approaching death, to Condronchi, seems very much in accord with the highest concerns for the patient and "to the sick more useful" (*aegrotanti utilius*), for a Christian will make more prudent use of remaining time. "Therefore, it is of enormous interest to the sick to know that he will die of his illness; and we should not listen to Galen who, since he was a pagan, extorts to audacity and rashness when he says that the physician although despairing about the health of the sick should always promise recovery."[51] We saw earlier that Castro, in many instances a true Galenist in temper (but of course writing and practicing in the Protestant city of Hamburg), in his discussion of simulation was about as daring on this issue. At the end of the period of my interest, Paolo Zacchia (1584–1659), after carefully reviewing the different shades of opinion of Renaissance doctors of medicine and canon law, daringly but with considerable trepidation arrives at this opinion:

> Thus I say that it does not seem to pertain to the physician to inform the sick in any way of his death except when clearly asked about it by this very patient, as it happens, at a particular moment out of concern for the welfare of his soul, or when there is no other way of avoiding a great scandal after the patient's death; in which latter case it may suffice to inform him through someone else.[52]

The other person may be a priest, confessor, or next of kin. Zacchia's medical justification is that otherwise the patient may fly into a rage (*ira*) against the doctor and worsen more quickly. This reasoning goes one step further than, for instance, Giovanni Colle (1558–1630), who advised that the physician should "cautiously" (*caute*) reveal that the disease is serious.[53] According to Zacchia, the physician on the one hand should not promise recovery when there is some danger of death, since the expectation of health might distract from the desire for eternal well-being, but on the other he should not (except for unusually compelling reasons, as mentioned above) announce to the patient that he will certainly die of his disease. The statement is important because (as is also evident in some rare early seventeenth-century instances, for example, in issues relating to abortion) the ethical duty of the physician is clearly seen as distinct and different from the ethical duty of others in charge of the spiritual and material welfare of the patient, and this in a work by a Roman Catholic published at Rome with all the requisite licenses and imprimatur.

If we look forward beyond the Renaissance and to the late eighteenth century, to Thomas Percival's important *Medical Ethics*, we find
that concern for the patient's soul has ceased to be a topic (at least in
Manchester, England), except that in a general sense Percival thinks
that "the *moral* and *religious* influence of sickness is . . . favourable to
the best interests of men and society."[54] According to Percival, a surgeon ought to give the surgical patient "assurance, if consistent with
truth, that the operation goes well" (p. 21). While no context is given
to justify outright lying, some dissimulation or silence about expected
deterioration of a patient's state of health is recommended: "A physician should not be forward, to make gloomy prognostications,
because they savour of empiricism, by magnifying the importance of
his services in the treatment of disease" (p. 31).

The Physician and the Adstantes

By *adstantes*, a word often used in Renaissance medical books, I mean
not just literally the persons standing about the sickbed, but the
world surrounding the patient and its concerns. Renaissance medical
authors realized that the problem of truth and falsehood does not
apply only to the physician's relation to the sick person but also to his
designs on the outside world.

To clarify the distinction, we may return to Elisha's message
(through Hazael) to King Ben-hadad of Syria that he shall recover.
(At the same time Elisha tells Hazael, the messenger, that God has
told him that the king shall surely die and that God has showed him
that Hazael will succeed to the throne.) We saw that Jakobovits uses
Elisha's lie to illustrate the Judaic value of relief for suffering over telling the sufferer the truth. The interpreter thus isolates one relationship out of the multiplicity of relationships represented in the triangle
above. If we go beyond the one verse reporting Elisha's message (2
Kings 8:10 or 4 Reg 8:10), the other relationships become saliently
obvious. For Elisha is very little concerned with the Syrian king's
health or well-being. Elisha weeps because he foresees that Hazael,
who he predicts will succeed Ben-hadad, will be the scourge of Israel.
Elisha's direction to say that the king may recover from the illness
though he forecasts the king's death probably indicates his knowledge that Hazael will tell him. In any case, all Elisha's words
(including the lie [*mendacium*] that, as the famous Renaissance exegete Cornelius a Lapide puts it, he seems to command Hazael to

utter) are directed at Hazael and show Elisha's design on him. In fact, the Renaissance commentator says about the effect of Elisha's words that Hazeal would be king of Syria: "Made more daring by this prediction of reigning, Hazael strangled the king and took over his kingdom."[55]

It hardly needs demonstration that the Renaissance for a number of reasons (many having to do with the inheritance of title and property) was acutely aware of the dimension I am highlighting now. In fact, some of the passages I cite show these concerns very clearly. The story Cortesi tells of a colleague's deceitful procedures (with which I opened my remarks on "The Physician and His Colleagues") is a case in point. This unscrupulous physician had lied when he predicted his female patient's quick recovery, as he admitted when citing Plato in his defense. What seems to irk Cortesi particularly in this doctor's behavior is not only that he had maligned his colleagues but that he had led the patient's husband to a wrong course of action (the dispatching of letters to relatives speaking of imminent cure) and that he thus had managed to discredit the medical profession.

Perhaps it needs to be said that classical warnings against treating the incurable are evidence not so much of a lack of charity as of worries about the ethics and hence reputation of the medical profession, pitched to high degree. In the passage adduced above, when Galen recommends that the physician promise certain recovery to an exceptionally fearful or troubled patient, he adds that the persons taking care of the sick ought to be told the truth.[56] Giovanni Colle (1558– 1630) in his *Cosmitor medicaeus* is considerably less precise than Galen or Celsus in this matter, but quite in tune with the ancient physicians' concerns about reputation when he recommends that "with a happy face and friendly look, the physician should give the patient and the *adstantes* hope, but sometimes, in order to vindicate himself from calumnies, he should immediately and cautiously state that the illness is serious."[57]

If the classical texts speak to the need of deceiving the patient in the interest of cure but not the *adstantes*, Renaissance texts occasionally advocate bending the truth somewhat even in respect to them. The following quotation represents practical advice to his students by Pietro Castelli (ca. 1590–1661), professor first at Rome and then at Messina, whose *Optimus medicus* I adduced earlier. The committed apologist of Hippocrates and distinguished botanist, in his work *Visitation of the Sick: For the Instruction of His Auditors and Students in*

Praxis, ranges from medical prudence, praised since Hippocrates, to a seemingly self-serving Machiavellianism, to which later writers on medical ethics (like Percival) reacted negatively:

> Therefore the physician will always say to the *adstantes* that the illness requires utmost attention and is most difficult (although it may at first appear light, because sometimes the serpent is lurking in the grass) and remedies need to be applied with great care. For if he thus has said that the disease is indeed serious, difficult to cure by others, he is hoping that it should be cured by his diligence and the patient's obedience. Thus if the patient regains his health, this will be attributed to the physician's diligence and knowledge; if he should die, then the physician will seem to have foreseen that correctly because of the seriousness of the disease. But if he should have said that the disease was minor (while it may be serious), he will gain no praise from the patient's recovery, since the illness, as he had put it, was minor. If he should then die, it will be the physician's fault, who would have been wrong both in his diagnosis and prognosis. Should the patient be in serious danger, in order not to come upon him deceased, and be made a laughing-stock, he will send an assistant to find out whether the patient is still alive. If he should unexpectedly come upon him deceased, he will rightaway say that he had foreknown that, but had come to learn at what hour the patient had died. I myself have seen young physicians easy and quick in their prognosis, but learned and old men very difficult, most ambiguous, and general. Hence you will understand me.[58]

But even this candor (approaching cynicism) toward future professionals had an antecedent in the Middle Ages, namely concern for the reputation of the profession: for the central recommendation— that the physician should lie about the purpose of his visit when discovering the patient dead (saying he came to ask the hour of death)— is in Arnald of Villanova.[59] The ubiquitous insistence in the Renaissance on the duty to inform the *adstantes* truthfully if the patient's condition is serious or desperate is a distant reflection of classical concerns about reputation. Thus Mercurialis (1530–1606) requires the physician to reveal the seriousness of the disease to relatives and *adstantes* in order to avoid scandal, a view with which Zacchia seems to agree, although he so clearly and courageously disagrees with some other Catholic physicians when he stresses that preserving the patient's peace of mind justifies not revealing it to the patient.[60]

From Cortesi's report and similar comments, we can tell that the "scandal" imagined is at least twofold: deception of the *adstantes* would indirectly result in calumny directed against the physician (as is spelled out by Giovanni Colle,[61] and the deceit would add to the disruption, in the family and larger society, caused by the patient's death. Apparently this latter aspect, the unpreparedness of society around the patient, is the *magnum scandalum* which Zacchia has in mind. As we saw in the passage I quoted, he takes this issue so seriously that its importance may, in special cases, override the other principle valued highly by him, namely keeping the patient at ease and confident in the ability of his physician. Of course, dynastic or political examples of the application of these principles abound. For the Renaissance, one might think of the hectic atmosphere around Queen Elizabeth's sickbed when she suffered from smallpox in October 1562 and was expected to die. (It is said that the Queen was too delirious to name her successor.[62]) A grotesque illustration of the rights of the *adstantes* to have the truth confirmed is President Lyndon Johnson's pulling up his shirt to show journalists the scars left from his gallbladder operation.

The reasoning about avoidance of a *scandalon*, which we see Zacchia applying in this context, is of course an important procedure in the (Roman Catholic) moral casuistry of the period, and had its place in evaluating claims of the world of the *adstantes*, which sometimes appear as the pressures of a patient's immediate society. The reasoning was applied to a problem that to any reader of *La Celestina* will not seem arcane, namely the question whether the physician may collaborate in pretending that his patient is a virgin. How to determine virginity, or rather the difficulty if not impossibility of establishing it, is frequently discussed in Renaissance medical literature. Sometimes the topic is discussed in contexts that by their title show their filiation from Galen's *Quomodo morbum simulantes sint deprehendi libellus* (Kühn ed. vol. 19). Thus in his book *De iis qui morbum simulant deprehendis*, Giovanni Battista Selvatico [d. 1621] expands on Galen by analyzing motives (primarily fear and gain) and then discussing in individual chapters various diseases and conditions commonly simulated or concealed: people simulate other diseases to hide pregnancies or syphilis; they pretend to be sterile or to be suffering from "retention of the menses" (for reasons we will discuss in a later chapter); and they pretend to be virgins.[63]

But the physician's collaboration in such deception poses a thorny ethical problem. Thus Juan-Alonso de los Ruyzes de Fontecha (1560–1620), after first mentioning some devices that might deceive the bridegroom into believing that he was rupturing a sound hymen (for instance, use of a gallbladder of a fish), says: "The doubt first arises whether without danger of conscience the physician can grant the woman requesting it that kind of help. For in truth what she requests is to deceive some man. But it is not right for men to deceive women either, as for instance, to seduce women."[64] Then Fontecha launches into the detailed exposition of the double nature of *dolus* in scholastic thought, summarized above. He adds that he had just such a request from a young woman once and proceeds to tell us the three steps he took to resolve his dilemma: (1) He went to a theologian (*vir theologus* and doctor of both laws) for advice, who thought the physician could participate in the deception if, and only if, by the device some great scandal would be avoided, i.e. if this woman were about to make public how she had been betrayed. (2) He consulted the diocesan *regens* and *moderator* of the committee on Holy Scripture (*posposci a D. de la Camera Sacrae Scripturae cathedrae moderatore, et gerente*), according to whom the physician was justified in helping her if he was confident that the woman wanted to be married and wanted to avoid causing herself and her family to suffer utter shame if she might appear spoiled to her groom. But if he thought that she was merely trying to pass herself off as a virgin without being one, he was not allowed to collaborate. (3) He asked the renowned theologian and moral casuist Vazquez, who agreed with the second opinion.

Fontecha, who held a chair of medicine at the University of Alcalá, wrote this book for beginning students of medicine, an introduction (or textbook, as we would say) to medicine and its ethics. Possibly by his detailed reasoning on this case he wanted to show his students the resources of which a physician should avail himself. If so, he may be taken to represent a perhaps typically Spanish and, in some sense, conservative approach to medical ethics, different from the one of which we have seen incipient signs in Zacchia: for the specialists to whom Fontecha resorts for advice are all moral casuists, i.e. theologians, not medical doctors, whereas Zacchia dared to reason specifically as a physician. In fact, for Fontecha, a distinction of these roles does not seem conceivable: toward the end of the discussion of the *casus* for which he has sought such detailed advice, he reveals that the woman has spoken to him "under the seal of confession ... and in his role of confessor" (*sub sigillo confessionis ... et medio confessore*), an important point in his reasoning only in so far as it rules out the possibility of *dolus malus*, a bad ruse, on her part. For some Renaissance physicians are acutely aware of the possibility of becoming themselves the victims of deceit, particularly in matters relating to sexual habits. (Citing Jason Pratensis [1486–1558], Meibom thus warns the physician against some clever women who might request him to write a prescription for some medication, for instance a strong purgative, for a patient that is absent—implying that they will use it on themselves to provoke an abortion.)[65] I should point out that in observing the unity of moral and medical ethics and calling this unity conservative, I may be revealing my bias as a modern historian. Fontecha ultimately relies on ecclesiastical authority, which in many aspects of life was repressive. *Conservative* here does not mean "preserving tradition," since his approach bespeaks that greatly intensified religious morality which may be the characteristic of the period in both Catholic and Protestant regions.

By any standards, Fontecha would have to be thought compassionate, but not quite as indulgent as François Ranchin, writing a few years later on the same subject. Ranchin, an often quoted medical authority and chancellor of the University of Montpellier, expressly reasoned as a physician. In his *Tractatus de morbis virginum*, Ranchin addresses the topic which, as he says, may seem dishonorable (*turpis*) to a physician but needs to be included for the sake of charity, in a subsection entitled, "The Repairing of Lost Virginity" (*De corruptae virginitatis reparatione*). For sometimes, he reasons, the physician has to collaborate in such *reparatio* for the honor of the young women and the future peace among spouses that otherwise might be uncertain. "Moreover, since such services are secret, I don't see by what reason they can be condemned. It is the duty of physicians to correct the weaknesses and defects of the parts of the body; but penitence of former sin with the desire to live properly is the concern of the theologians and the girls themselves."[66]

It might seem that rather than being evidence of a sense of distinction between medical ethics and other forms of moral casuistry, these sentences are evidence that Ranchin washes his hands of ethical questions altogether, but this would be mistaken. Not only does he frequently express ethical judgement, but his views are often and seriously considered by such writers as Zacchia and Boudewyns, the latter of whom, at the end of the period of my interest, collects and integrates his predecessors' statements on medical ethics. In fact, after the sentence I just quoted, Ranchin goes on to say that the controlling motive in his action (to veil sins by "repairing" virginity) is the virtue of prudence, and that such medical action should not encourage others to license. From his very first sentence on the subject Ranchin indicates that he is dealing with a controversial subject that touches the reputation of his profession. Therefore, his spelling out what he considers the duties of the physician in the secrecy of medical consultation is a conscious act, perhaps a minor milestone in the history of medical ethics.

It hardly needs pointing out that dialectically the notion of secrecy, while screening off the relationship to the *adstantes*, confirms it. Renaissance medical authors frequently mention the physician's duty to keep knowledge about the patient's infirmities secret, in Catholic areas, understandably with reference to the duties of confessors. Thus, discussing the Hippocratic oath, Meibom (who is a Protestant) quotes Louis Lobera d'Avila (fl. 1530) in Italian as saying: "The physician should be diligent, studious, of good conscience, honest, and discrete as a confessor."[67] Meibom then proceeds to give a very detailed and thoughtful summary of Renaissance opinion on the limits of this right to secrecy, summarizing the views of the celebrated moral casuist Azor (who is not a physician) that the physician need not reveal information gained in confidence (since this "natural right" to be silent supersedes other laws), but also the physician Valleriola's insistence that the government has a right to be informed about contagious diseases.[68]

After considering these matters of openness and secrecy, closely related to the thread of truth/falsehood that I have been following, we are now ready to return to the case reported by Fortunato Fidele that introduced this chapter. Fidele reports:

> I knew a girl in her flourishing youth, who consulted her physician about aborting a fetus before its time. In order to foil her undertaking, the physician, in a pious misrepresentation (*pia simulatione*), promised her he would give her something that would fulfill her expectation entirely: but in truth he mixed an antidote from ingredients that should make the fetus strong and healthy. However, the girl had hardly drunk it down, when she

began to burn with the desire to bring forth, and hoping that what she had been promised falsely would certainly happen, entirely bent on this one concern, she before long felt the fetus had dropped down; and to the disgrace (*ignominia*) of the physician, she aborted in spite of the resisting medication. For the image of the abortion, so strongly conceived, both overcame the power of the medication and foiled the physician's endeavor.

This case illustrates at least four important categories that we lifted from the many possible ones in medical ethics: (1) the relationship of one doctor to another, for it is told (according to the section title) by a doctor evaluating errors of judgment of his colleagues. Since by its nature, details of the case originate from the physician whose professional reputation is at stake, there is at least the possibility of deception. (2) If we read the case the way Fidele intended it to be read and accept the surface sense, which is undoubtedly the safer procedure, the working of this *pharmakon* is a striking example of the powers of the imagination, as the Renaissance conceived them. I have argued elsewhere that in Montaigne (who wrote most memorably on this subject) and others, the strongest manifestations of these powers tend to be conceived negatively, i.e. as interfering with the proper functioning and performance of the human body,[69] and this case of an abortion possibly reflects such notions. From a slightly different perspective, if we could give full credit to the report that the medication produced an effect exactly opposite to its ordinary use, it would be the ultimate of cases illustrating the imagination's effect on the body, more striking perhaps than even Fienus's extraordinary variety. (3) In modern terms it would demonstrate powerfully the placebo effect of medicine. Thus the case is also related to the *fiducia* problems mentioned above. As in the other contexts where we found *fiducia* discussed in the Renaissance, the effect of the patient's trust in the physician is powerfully shown, but the other side, the physician's obligation in this relationship, is only partially expressed. This is so even though the physician's procedure is criticized by the medical author. In his introductory sentences, which I did not translate, Fidele warns physicians not to collaborate in any abortion and not even to give remedies to pregnant women that might raise their expectation of help. Although he thus condemns deceit in this case, the issue is never addressed as a deontological problem, as an injunction to the physician to be truthful to his patient. But his warning against promising help that will not be given is no less interesting for having the specifics of Renaissance medical theory (the particular powers of the imagination in pregnant women), i.e., for remaining a very specific medical problem. (4) The *adstantes*, the society around patient and physician, are represented in the reported case by the narrator (who we may assume heard of the case as forensic investigator) and possibly also by the moral pressures that make the physician want to foil the girl's intent and most clearly by the "institution" dispensing *ignominia*.

With all this richness of reference, Fidele's case at the most only indirectly questions the physician's right to simulate: after all, the particular physician's *simulatio* was characterized as *pia*, his intention honorable. If the case is presented to illustrate poor practice or even malpractice, it is because the physician ignored the power of the imagination and in a strange way reversed or even perverted the use of simulation for the purposes of curing.

Results

As I look back at my aspirations and aims as I entered into this topic, I am humbled by my results. Impressed by the clarity of that moment in the history of ethics represented by Kant's disagreement with Benjamin Constant, I wanted to project their positions backward and find their ancestors in Protestant/Puritan and Catholic/moral casuist ethical divisions. I also had in mind Pascal's famous ridicule (in the *Provinciales*) of (the Jesuits') moral casuistry as he saw it from his radical Augustinian position. His mocking charge was that his Jesuit opponent had discussed whether it was a greater sin for a priest to visit a house of prostitution in disguise or wearing his *soutane*, but had not addressed the fundamental issue that the priest should not go there at all. There may be a number of reasons why I failed to find the positions of Kant and Constant prefigured clearly in the medical ethics of the Renaissance. (1) There are many more books of cases and medical letters, etc., to screen. I may not have looked long enough. (2) I may have looked in the wrong places. By limiting myself to "rational" medicine, I excluded dozens of Paracelsian medical works, many of them written by radical Protestants. Paracelsian works are quite different, often beginning with the requirement of high ethics and godliness in the medical practitioner or, rather, "priest-physician" (as Peter Elmer has pointed out[70]), and rarely work down to the level of medical casuistry. (3) In addition to this difficulty of defining a body of Protestant medical books (from which to derive a Protestant medical ethics), the issue is further complicated by the fact that some of the most distinguished writers on this subject who practiced and published for decades in Protestant cities were Portuguese Jews who had received their medical training in Spain (Rodrigo a Castro of Hamburg and Abraham Zacutus of Amsterdam). The next chapter will be devoted to them. (4) This part of the problem may be ill conceived, since the area in which I hoped to see reflections of the larger disagreement is medical casuistry, and it may be claimed that any kind of casuistry, whether legal, moral, or medical, will show how poorly general laws fit practice, and thus demonstrate an un-Kantian compromise and adjustment. From this point of view, it may be significant that Calvin's Protestant opponent on the issue of simulation in religious matters, the adversary representing the position labeled "Nicodemist," was a former monk turned physician, Otto Brunfels (1488–1534), although I have not found anything particularly telling in the *medical* works by Brunfels available to me.[71]

Some related questions remain and have perhaps become more pressing for me: Can it be an accident that the physicians I identified as being the most resourceful in devising stratagems to cure "melancholics" hail from Spain or received their medical training in Spain, home of some of the foremost moral casuists? (Zacuto had been a student at the famous University of Salamanca.) In other words, is there some link, however "deep," in the structure of thinking between moral casuistry, in which so many Jesuits distinguished themselves, and the justification of this particular therapy? (For students of imaginative literature, this question is of some consequence, since the desire to satirize ingenious attempts at curing Don Quixote animates much of Cervantes' famous novel.) But at present, while the relationship of that same moral casuistry to medicine and the then emerging thinking about medical ethics remains largely uncharted, it would seem foolhardy for me to suggest answers to such a specific question. In the next chapter, we will take up one strand of this complex of problems by focusing more specifically on the contribution to medical ethics of physicians who were "Lusitani," which almost invariably means expatriate Jews from Portugal, educated on the Iberian peninsula, usually in Spain. Castro, whose *Medicus-Politicus* was written for the senate of Hamburg, in that work praises the thoughtfulness of the Spanish medical curriculum of which he had been a beneficiary and

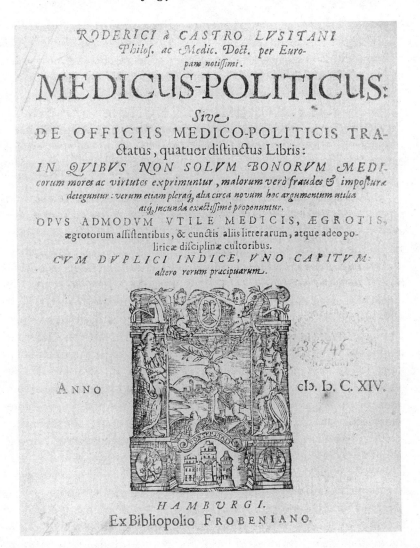

RODERICI à CASTRO LVSITANI
Philof. ac Medic. Doct. per Euro-
pam notiſſimi.

MEDICUS-POLITICUS:

Sive

DE OFFICIIS MEDICO-POLITICIS TRA-
ctatus, quatuor diſtinctus Libris:

IN QVIBVS NON SOLVM BONORVM MEDI-
corum mores ac virtutes exprimuntur, malorum verò fraudes & impoſturæ
deteguntur: verum etiam pleraq, alia circa novum hoc argumentum utilia
atq, jncunda exactiſſimè proponuntur.

OPVS ADMODVM VTILE MEDICIS, ÆGROTIS,
ægrotorum aſſiſtentibus, & cunctis aliis litterarum, atque adeo po-
liricæ diſciplinæ cultoribus.

CVM DVPLICI INDICE, VNO CAPITVM:
altero rerum præcipuarum.

ANNO   cIↄ. Iↄ. C. XIV.

HAMBVRGI.
Ex Bibliopolio FROBENIANO.

Figure 2.1. Frontispiece of Rodrigo a Castro, *Medicus-Politicus*, Hamburg, 1614 (National Library of Medicine).

compares it favorably with medical training in Germany. In this context one wonders whether Castro was expressing more than a conventional *topos modestiae* when he called his *Medicus-Politicus* a mere *lusus*
(entertainment, sport). Was he adopting the perspective of some German critics (as opposed to Zacuto, who praised the work to the sky),

to whom this area of interest, medical ethics, seemed unserious? Certainly later medical historians showed a contemptuous disregard for this branch of human endeavor in their concentration on only those elements of medicine that lead to, or prefigure, modern medicine as a "hard" science. As I mentioned before, August Hirsch's biographical dictionary of medical doctors, assembled in the late nineteenth century but several times reprinted and still used as one of the major research tools for the history of medicine, calls all of Meibom's publications "insignificant" and considers Boudewyns's *Ventilabrum medico theologicum* second rate.[72]

Although particular elements of my hypothesis remain unproven, the area in which medical ruse, pretense, or lie is discussed and opposed to truthfulness has turned out to be most revealing. While the issue of medical pretense in the interest of curing appears hallowed by some classical approval, theoretically minded physicians like Cortesi and Castro make truthfulness (and its opposite) the subject of extensive inquiries, to which they devote entire chapters. Their answer makes use of the tools of moral casuistry and, in the frequent emphasis on consideration for the *adstantes*, explicates classical interests in the reputation and self-validation of the medical profession at large. In Renaissance discussions of the crucial Platonic passage we noticed attempts at defusing it medically by moving it into the area of political power, where the Renaissance may have accepted as commonplace a degree of deceit by the ruler, i.e. of what is loosely called Machiavellianism. At the same time, many physicians saw value in "simulation" for good ends, as in the story of Hagnodice, the woman who is said to have deceived her (male) colleagues in order to practice medicine and serve the particular needs of female patients.

In the relationship of the physician to his colleagues the topic of falsehood/pretense versus truth is frequently articulated as a warning against the practitioner who is ignorant or a fraud, and such warnings are addressed to other colleagues, to the civic authorities (as in the case of Castro), or even to the patient. In doctor-patient relationships, the stories presenting the devices to cure cases of melancholy are mainstays of the medical literature of the period. Two of the paradigms within which I saw these cases are only implicit in that period: resourcefulness (implied in the word *artificium*) and roughness versus gentleness (the latter implied in the word *socius*, a companion or friend who will join the patient and pretend to suffer from a similar condition). The third was explicitly a concern at the time, and we should be careful not to dismiss it as a philosophical rather than medical issue. For to argue and "prove" that the mind cannot cure the body (except *accidentally*, as Fienus put it, following scholastic uses of speech) was firing a powerful blast at "empirical" and even Paracelsian medicine and its reliance on murky, dark, poorly understood phenomena, in short, the magical. The line of argument emphasized here confirms the differentiation Brian Vickers argued most persuasively for related areas of knowledge and seems contiguous also with Peter Elmer's questioning of what has been called the "puritanism-science" hypothesis. Other than in such questions of spiritual effects, discussions of the power of *fiducia* follow ancient precedent: they stress the importance of the patient's trust in the ability of the physician and sometimes show how the physician sought, even at times grotesquely, to add what we may call a placebo effect to his medication, as by giving it a Punic name. That Galeotto Marzio does so uncritically indicates that *fiducia* was taken to be only the confidence located in the patient and that the physician-patient relationship was rarely conceived in the legal sense of fiduciary (commentaries on a few well-known prescriptions in the Hippocratic oath are the exception).

Since for a number of reasons (including, of course, the feudal and patriarchal nature of society), female virginity was extraordinarily prized if not fetishized, the role of the physician in relation to this topic is addressed in a number of Renaissance medical works. I concentrated on two medical authors who chose different resolutions for the dilemma of the physicians caught between the demands of patient and society. Rather than evaluating their solutions—both are very thoughtful—I am of course interested in the different ways they went about solving their problem. Unquestionably these passages were intended to be models for the writers' colleagues and students: Fontecha resorted to experts in moral theology, the expert "ethics" available to him, while Ranchin contrasted the role of the physician with that of the theologian and derived his ethics from the function of the physician as he saw it. Although I emphasized the difference between their solutions, which is significant, the physicians share a keen interest in the ethical dilemmas of a doctor. If we should cast our net wider, we would find that while the topic of true and pretended virginity looms large, not all writers focus on questions of ethical conduct of the physician. Thus, in his *Medicus-Politicus*, Castro avoids the dilemma by adopting the forensic perspective, namely of how to recognize pretense if the physician is called upon as arbiter; this assumes that the physician is siding with the *adstantes*, i.e. society. But it would be foolish to try to contrast on these narrow grounds a personal medical ethics of Montpellier with a state hygienics of Hamburg.

At the same time, Ranchin's carving out of an area of medical ethics in which the moral theologian has no say is important. Although as a rhetorical move it can be linked with some of Galen's strategies, in the context of Renaissance France it was daring. We saw that a little later Zacchia (writing at Rome, of all places) adopts the same procedure as he discusses the question whether the physician should tell the incurably ill the truth. I suspect that these moments of medical moral analysis, which could be multiplied if we included other traditional topics of ethical contention (for instance abortion), are milestones in the history of medical ethics. It cannot be an accident that in both these "moments" the physicians seemed to side with Plato, according to whom falsehood was useful as a *pharmakon*, rather than with Aristotle (or the intransigent Kant). In various particular situations, both Ranchin and Zacchia would have said, with Julius Alexandrinus, *mentiamur sane*, let us lie healthily.

NOTES

1. Fortunato Fidele, *De relationibus medicorum* (Palermo, 1602), lib. 2, c. 10, sectio "De physicorum erroribus iudicandis," p. 184: "Puellam novi, florenti aetate: quae cum de foete ante tempus abijciendo (sic) medicum consuleret: hic ut impium illius institutum falleret, pia simulatione promittit, se daturum quidem, quod suam expectationem abunde expleret: verum antidotum ex iis miscuit, quae foeti robur, ac firmitudinem adjicerent: Puella tamen dum illo hausto, iam tum pariendi desiderio vehementer incensa esset, ac certo sibi, quod falso promittebatur, eventurum sperans, tota in hanc curam incumbens, non multo post elapsum esse foetum sensit: ac, non sine medici ignominia abortivit pharmaco quantumlibet adversante: nam vehemens illa abortus concepta imago, et medicamenti vim vicit, et medici operam elusit."

2. Carera, *Le confusioni de medici. Opera nella quale si scuopono gl'errori, e gl'inganni de Medici* (Milano, 1652), p. 162: ". . . la vera definitione dall'Arte Medica era questa *Medicina est Ars illudendi Mundum, et a qua totus Mundus delusus est.*"

3. Littré ed., vol. 4, p. 639.

4. "Über ein vermeintliches Recht aus Menschenliebe zu lügen," in Kant, *Werke* (Frankfurt: Suhrkamp, 1968): vol. 8, pp. 637–43.

5. Zagorin, *Ways of Lying: Dissimulation, Persecution, and Conformity in Early Modern Europe* (Cambridge, Mass., and London: Harvard Univ. Press,

1990), particularly chap. 4; "Calvinism and Nicodemism;" Carlo Ginzburg, *Il nicodemismo: Simulazione e dissimulazione religiosa nell'Europa del '500* (Torino: Einaudi, 1970).

6. See D. von Engelhardt, "Geburt und Tod—medizinethische Betrachtungen in historischer Perspective," in *Anfang and Ende des menschlichen Lebens: Medizinethische Probleme*, ed. O. Marquard and H. Staudinger (Paderborn: Schöningh, 1987), p. 63.

7. *Fori medici adumbratio* (Coberg, 1607).

8. Bk. 3, 329B; Loeb ed., vol. 1, p. 213. See also Jacques Derrida's far-ranging discussion of Plato's use of the word *pharmakon* in other works, *La dessémination* (Paris: Seuil, 1972).

9. Rodrigo a Castro, *Medicus-Politicus*, (Hamburg, 1614), chap. 9: "Liceatne medico aegrum fallere valetudinis gratia," p. 142.

10. Hippocrates, *In epidem.* 6, sec. 5.7 (or 5.13) and sec. 4.7 or 4.8 (ed. Littré, vol. 5, pp. 319 and 309); for Galen's commentary on these passges, i.e. the ruse and the passage on "gratifying" patients or "accommodating" oneself to them, see Kühn ed., vol. 17, par. 2, pp. 266–69 and 135–43, or Galen, *Omnia quae exstant* (Basel, 1561), tertia classis, pp. 374–75 and 353–55; for telling the "prudent" patient the truth, but lying to the fearful (*timidus*), see Galen, Kühn ed., vol. 17, par. 1, pp. 995–96. In well-annotated editions of the Hippocratic corpus, as in the Frankfurt edition of 1595, Castro would have found Galen's commentary integrated into the elaborate annotations to the text. See Hippocrates, *Opera omnia quae extant* (Frankfurt, 1595), VII, pp. 279 and 282 (for the earache episode and commentary on it) and VII, pp. 273 and 275.

11. Castro, *Medicus-Politicus*, p. 143: "Et quidem Hipp. *in Epidemiis* sapius deceptionem suadere videatur, et Galenus addit aliquando falso esse adjicienda."

12. Theodore Zwinger, *Theatrum humanae vitae* (Basel, 1604), p. 2849, where the distinction is based on Aristotle: "Simulationem enim Aristoteles proprie tribuit excessui veritatis, Dissimulationem defectui. Simulans, id quod non est, esse fingit: Dissimulans, id quod est, non esse fingit." My impression is that even the moral casuists were not consistent in distinguishing the two, and it may be telling that Perez Zagorin, author of the most recent and reliable study of the phenomenon of dissimulation in early modern Europe, does not make that distinction in his own discourse either.

13. Darrel Amundsen notes the interest in the curative effect of confession in the relevant documents, particularly the canon of 1215 bearing the incipit *Cum infirmitas* (or *Quuminfirmitas*). See "Casuistry and Professional Obligations: The Regulation of Physicians by the Court of Conscience in the Late Middle Ages—Part II," *Transactions and Studies of the College of Physicians of Philadelphia*, 5th ser., vol. 3 (1981), pp. 93–112 (particularly pp. 96–97).

14. Castro, *Medicus-Politicus* p. 142: "Alia enim est simulatio, qua veritas tacendo subtrahitur, aut quovis velamine circumtegitur: alia, qua falsus pro vero exprimitur. Prima non modo inculpabilis, quinimo suo loco et tempore digna laude virtusque reputanda censetur."

15. Ibid.; Galen, *De methodo medendi*, 14.16 (Kühn ed., vol. 10, p. 1009).

16. Castro, *Medicus-Politicus* p. 143: "Sic ostentatio ignito cauterio uterus collapsus ad suam sedem saepe reducitur: et in extremis malis non videtur abs re, aliud sentire, aliud loqui, ne ad desperationem adigatur infirmus."

17. See, for example, Baptista Codronchi, *De Christiana ac tuta medendi ratione* (Ferrara, 1591), p. 146.

18. *Medicus-Politicus*, p. 145: "Verum haec exempla divinioris altiorisque sunt contemplationis ac secretioris sensus." On the background of such discussions of lying, particularly Augustine's *Against Lying* (where such cases of dissimulation are treated as prophetic, mystical, or "figurative"), see Zagorin, *Ways of Lying*, chap. 2, "Sources," particularly pp. 21–24.

19. Giovanni Battista Cortesi, *Miscellaneorum medicinalium decades* (Messanae, 1625), decas 10, quaestio 6, pp. 763–64.

20. Plato, *Opera Omnia*, trans. Ficino (Frankfurt, 1602) pp. 602–09.

21. "*Tractatus quatuor distinctis libris: in quibus non solum bonorum medicorum mores ac virtutes exprimuntur malorum vero fraudes et imposturae deteguntur.*"

22. Castelli, *Optimus medicus* (Messanae, 1637), p. 2: "Simillimi enim huiusmodi Medici sunt personis, quae tragoediis introducuntur; quemadmodum enim illi figuram quidem, et habitum, ac personam eorum quos referunt habent, illi ipsi autem vere non sunt: sic et Medici fama quidem et nomine multi, re autem, et opere valde pauci."

23. Johann Heinrich Meibomius, *Horkos, sive jusjurandum* (Leyden, 1643), p. 149.

24. Ambroise Paré, *De la chirurgie*, liv. 1, c. 30 in *Oeuvres* (4th ed., Paris, 1585), p. LIV.

25. *The Key to Unknown Knowledge* (London, 1599), sig. I 4ᵛ.

26. Codronchi, *De Christiana ac tuta medendi ratione* (Ferrara, 1591), lib. 1, c. 37, p. 112: ". . . si necessitas cogat eos vocare ubi videlicet christiani Medici desint, sive non satis apti et positi ad illius morbi curationem." The chapter is entitled programmatically: "Medicus adhibens sibi socium in curationibus Iudaeum vel alius ad medendum advocans, vel medicamenta ab eis accipens exceptis quibusdam casibus peccat."

27. Ranchin, *Tractatus de consultationibus medicis*, in *Opuscula medica* (Lyon, p. 1627), p. 701.

28. Laurent Joubert, *Erreurs populaires au fait de la medicine et regime de santé* (Bordeaux, 1578), p. 248: "Touttefois nous leur quittons cette partie de la chirurgie, quant à l'anfantemant: parce qu'il est plus honeste que ce metier là se fasse de fame à fame ez parties honteuses. . . ."

29. *Medicorum ecclesiasticum diarium* (Louvain, 1595), p. 136.

30. Campbell Bonner, "The Trial of Saint Eugenia," *American Journal of Philology* 41 (1920): 260. Margaret Alic assumes the story to be historical, I do not know on what authority; see *Hypatia's Heritage: A History of Women from Antiquity to the Late Nineteenth Century* (London: Women's Press, 1986): pp. 28–30.

31. Girolamo Bardi, *Medicus politico Catholicus* (Genua, 1644), p. 278.

32. For the Latin version, see Hyginus, *Fabularum liber* (Basel 1535), where the story (no. 274) is on p. 63. For a modern translation see *The Myths of Hyginus*, trans. and ed. Mary Grant (Lawrence, Kans: University of Kansas Press, 1960), pp. 175–76.

33. Curiously, she was included in Johannes Molanus's calendar *Medicorum ecclesiasticum diarium* (Louvain, 1595), p. 39 (5 Feb.).

34. Alphonso Ponce de Santecruz, *Dignotio et cura affectuum melancholicorum* (Madrid, 1622), fol. 2.

35. Alexandrinus, *De medicina et medico* (Zürich, 1557), p. 334: "... mentiamur sane ... quando neque exercituum ducibus, neque principibus civitatum, turpe umquam fuit mentiri in civitatum, aut exercituum suorum salutem."

36. The literature on this subject is immense. I found most useful Harald Weinrich, *Das Ingenium Don Quijotes* (Forschungen zur Romanischen Philologie, Heft 1), Münster: Aschendorf, 1956. See also my essay "Renaissance Exempla of Schizophrenia: The Cure by Charity in Luther and Cervantes," *Renaissance and Reformation* n.s. 9 (1985): 157–76.

37. Abraham Zacuto, *De medicorum principum historia* in *Opera Omnia* (Lyon, 1642), lib. 1, observatio 39 (p. 75). I translated the following passages: "... quae ad insomniam, maciam, tristitiam factitari solent;" "At nos visis his prudenter, incassum tamen celebratis, alio artificio praesidio usi sumus;" "Melancholici ergo, si arte curari non possunt, industria, et fallacis opus est, quibus sanari experientia confirmat." Unquestionably, the cure sounds unbelievable only to us; the Renaissance appears to have abounded with divine voices, real and pretended. For a similar stratagem of pretending a divine pronouncement (through a hole made in a wall at Gray's Inn), see the story reported of young William Cecil, later Lord Burghley, by Conyers Read, *Mr. Secretary Cecil and Queen Elizabeth* (London: Cape, 1962), pp. 30–31.

38. This case and similar ones are reported in Luther's *Colloquia*. Castro has a whole group of play-actors dressed in white eating. See *Medicus-Politicus*, p. 161. I have discussed many such reports of cure in "Renaissance Exempla of Schizophrenia."

39. *Observationum libri tres* (Basel, 1614), pp. 40–43; see my essay "Justifying the Unjustifiable: The Dover Cliff Scene in *King Lear*," *Shakespeare Quarterly* 36 (1985): 337–43.

40. Santacruz, *Dignotio et cura affectuum melancholicorum* (Madrid, 1622), fol. 16: "Aperite (obsecro) amici mei et ... iam enim non vas vitreum, sec miserrimum omnium me iudico, praecipue si hic igne isto me vitam agere sinitis. Timor enim, ne flamma consumeretur, sic intensus fuit, ut causa esset abolitionis falsae imaginationis."

41. Zacuto, *De medicorum principum historia*, lib. 1, observatio 38, p. 75: "Sicque deposita imaginatione intra paucos dies sanus evasit."

42. Thomas Fienus, *De viribus imaginationis* (Leyden, 1635; 1st ed., 1608), quaestio M: *An possit [imaginatio] morbos curare?* p. 193: "Scribit Thomas à Vega quendam ex suis decumbentem causo frequenter in delirio obnixissime medicos rogasse, ut liceret sibi in illo stagno (pavimentum monstrabat) natare, dicendo quod exinde esset convaliturus: & medicos id ei tandem concessisse: illum tum se in pavimentum mox dejecisse, & cum in eo aliquanto tempore fuisset volutatus, cum summa laetitia dixisse, aquam nunc ad genua, & paulo altius ascendisse: & cum ultimo sibi persuaderet eam jam usque ad guttur pervenisse, dixisse, se jam sanum esse, & revera sanum evasisse."

43. See the chapter "Mind and Sense" in Nancy B. Siraisi, *Taddeo Alderotti and his Pupils: Two Generations of Italian Medical Learning* (Princeton, N.J.: Princeton University Press, 1981), pp. 203–236. Also Brian Vickers, "Analogy versus Identity: The Rejection of Occult Symbolism, 1580–1680," in *Occult and Scientific Mentalities in the Renaissance*, ed. Brian Vickers (Cambridge University Press, 1984), pp. 95–163. Charles Schmitt has written about regional variations of the conflict between Platonism and Aristotelianism; see his *The Aristotelian Tradition and Renaissance Universities* (London: Variorum Reprints, 1984), particularly essay no. xv.

44. *De doctrina promiscua* (Lyon, 1552).

45. For Ranchin, see *Pathologia universalis*, sec. 2, chap. 7 in *Opuscula medica*, p. 105; Charles B. Schmitt, "Philosophy and Science in Sixteenth-Century Italian Universities," in his *The Aristotelian Tradition and Renaissance Universities*, essay xv, particularly p. 315. Alexandrinus (or Alessandrini) defended Galen against the critique of Argenterio. Personal physician of two princes (Ferdinand I and Maximilian II), he died reputed to be an exceptional physician. As we shall see in chap. 3, Rodrigo a Castro used his book about the physician.

46. *De medicina et medico* (Zürich, 1557), p. 334–41.

47. Galeotto Marzio, *De doctrina promiscua*, p. 164: ". . . unde utilissimum est pro vulgo imperito Punica aut Graeca aut alia, omissa quae nota est, loqui."

48. Botallo, *Commentarioli duo, alter de medici, alter de aegroti munere* (Lyon, 1565), p. 31.

49. On the medieval history of these problems, see M. E. Graf Matuschka, "Ärztliche Deontologie im Mittelalter," *Die medizinische Welt* 37 (1986): 378–80, and Hans Schadewaldt, "Arzt und Patient in antiker und frühchristlicher Sicht," *Medizinische Klinik* 59 (1964), 146–52.

50. Entry "Judaism," *Encyclopedia of Bioethics* (New York and London, 1978), p. 798.

51. Giovanni Battista Codronchi, *De Christiana medendi ratione*, p. 58: "Quare aegroti per magni interest scire eo se morbo moritutum (sic); neque hoc loco audiendus est Gal. qui cum esset Ethnicus ad audaciam et temeritatem hortatur, ut scilicet Medicus, quamvis desperet de salute aegrotantis semper incolumitatem polliceatur."

52. Zacchia, *Quaestiones medico-legales* (Rome, 1634), lib. 6, titulus 1, quaestio 4 (p. 25): "Dico igitur, non videri ad Medicum pertinere mortem aliquo modo aegro nunciare nisi forte ab ipso aegro, ut fit, instanter ab suae animae salutem, de hoc interrogetur, aut si nulla alia via sit, qua magnum scandalum evitari post aegri mortem posset, licet sufficeret eo casu per alium hoc aegro denunciare."

53. *Cosmitor medicaeus* (Venice, 1621), p. 30. Educated at Padua, Colle practiced medicine in Venice for fifteen years before his reputation gained him a post at the court of the Duke of Urbino.

54. *Medical Ethics: A Code of Institutions and Precepts Adapted to the Professional Conduct of Physicians and Surgeons* (Manchester, 1803), pp. 11–12; first ed. 1794.

55. Cornelius a Lapide (van den Steen), *In libros Regum et Paralipomenon commentarius* (Paris, 1642), p. 430: "Hac regni praedictione audacior factus Hazaël regem Benadad suffocavit, eiusque regnum occupavit." It is of course interesting that, according to the Jesuit interpreter, Elisha only *seems* to command Hazael to use a lie. Cornelius a Lapide explains Elisha's *sanaberis* as *ex morbo hoc non morieris,* i.e. as a kind of equivocation.

56. Galen, Kühn ed., vol. 17, pars 1, 996.

57. *Cosmitor medicaeus,* pp. 29–30: ". . . laeta serenaque fronte, iucundoque aspectu spem afferat aegrotanti, et adstantibus, aliquando etiam, ut calumniis se vindicet prompte, et caute attestetur morbum gravem esse."

58. Castelli, *De visitatione aegrotantium. Pro suis auditoribus et discipulis ad praxim instruendis* (Rome, 1630), p. 80: "Dicat ergo semper Medicus Astantibus Morbum esse maxime considerationis, et difficultatis (licet primo appareat levis, quia aliquando Serpens latet in herba) et remedia cum multa diligentia esse adhibenda. si ergo dixerit morbus per se, esse quidem magnum, et ab aliis curatu difficilem, tamen sua diligentia, et aegri obedentia se sperare ipsum esse sanandum. ita si aeger recuperabit sanitatem diligentiae, et scientiae Medici tribuetur; si vero Mors accesserit, iam Medicum eam praevidisse ob morbi atrocitate, videbitur, si vero Medicus dixerit Morbum esse levem (qui sit magnus) si sanabitur, nil laudis acquiret, quia morbus, ut dixerat, erat levis. si moriatur aeger culpa erit Medici, quod non cognoverit Morbum nec recte praedixerit, et suo errore obiisse, quod si in extremis fuerit aeger, ne Medicus indicat in Mortuum, et irrideatur. mittat famulum, vel discipulum ad sciendum, an aeger vivat, quod si inscienter inciderit in defunctum. alacriter dicat se iam praescivisse, sed velle scire qua hora mortuus fuerit, et equidem testor me observasse iuvenes faciles in prognosticando. senes vero doctos difficillimos, et maxime ambiguos, et universales. vos igitur me intellexistis."

59. Arnald of Villanova (ca. 1240–1311), *De cautelis medicorum,* trans. Henry E. Sigerist: "If by hard luck you come to the home of the patient and find him dead and somebody perhaps says: 'Sir, what have you come for?' You shall say that you have not come for that, and say that you well knew that he was going to die that night but that you wanted to know at what hour he had died." From *A Source Book of Medieval Science,* ed. Edward Grant (Cambridge, Mass.: Harvard University Press, 1974), p. 752.

60. Zacchia cites Mercurialis, *Errorum popularium libri,* lib. 2, cap. 25, apparently in agreement. See Zacchia, *Quaestiones medico-legales,* lib. 6, tit. 1, quaestio 4 (p. 25).

61. *Cosmitor medicaeus,* p. 30: ". . . ut calumniis se vindicet . . ."

62. See Neville Williams, *Thomas Howard, Fourth Duke of Norfolk* (London: Barrie and Rockliff, 1964), p. 84.

63. Selvatico, *De iis qui morbum simulant deprehendis* (Milan, 1595). On virginity, see chap. 9.

64. *Medicorum incipientium medicina, sive medicinae Christianae speculum* ([Alcalá], 1598), p. 612: "Dub. tamen primum insurgit, an absque periculo conscientiae medicus mulieri ab eodem expostulanti hoc praesidium possit concedere: nam revera ut decipiat hominem aliquem, id quaerit: fallere autem mulieres homines non decet: sicuti nec homines seducere mulieres: esse vero illud dolum, insinuant omnes summistae. . . ."

65. *Horkos, sive jusjurandum*, p. 149.

66. Ranchin, *Tractatus de morbis virginum*, sec. 3, chap. 2 (p. 445), in his *Opuscula medica* "Addo quod cum secreta sint eiusmodi officia, non video qua ratione damnari possint. Medicorum munus est, partium corporis infirmitates, et defectus corrigere; poenitentia quidem peccati praeteriti cum desirio bene vivendi a Theologis, & a puellis spectanda."

67. Louis Lobera d'Avila, *Delle infermità cortegiane*, lib. 4, c. 27, quoted from Meibomius, *Horkos, sive jusjurandum*, p. 190: "Deve il Médico esser diligente, studiose, di buona conscienza, honesto, & secreto, come un confessore."

68. In addition to the many authors cited by Meibom (pp. 190–92), see on the subject Michel Boudewyns, *Ventilabrum medico-theologicum* (Antwerp, 1666), par. 1, quaestio 41 (pp. 247–54). The work by Azor is *Institutiones morales* (Rome, 1600–1606), 2 vols.

69. See my *Melancholy, Genius, and Utopia in the Renaissance* (Wiesbaden: Harrassowitz, 1991), pp. 178–181.

70. Peter Elmer, "Medicine, Religion, and the Puritan Revolution," in *The Medical Revolution of the Seventeenth Century*, ed. Roger French and Andrew Wear (Cambridge and New York: Cambridge University Press, 1989), pp. 10–45, particularly p. 16.

71. See Carlo Ginzburg, *Il nicodemismo: Simulazione e dissimulazione religiosa nell'Europa del '500*, p. xiv: "La prima formulazione della dottrina della liceità della simulazione si trova nei *Pandectarus veteris et novi Testamenti, libri xii* di Otto Brunfels, aparsi a Strasburgo nel 1527." Brunfels proposed the thesis that the true church is spiritual and that ceremonies therefore do not count, a position Ginzburg characterizes as "ecclesiologia 'spiritualistica'" (p. 53). Erich Sanwald's dissertation is helpful, but unfortunately the parts published focus on Brunfels's theology, omitting the chapters that deal with his life and career as a physician: *Otto Brunfels 1488–1535: Ein Beitrag zur Geschichte des Humanismus und der Reformation*, diss. München (Bottrop: Postberg, 1932).

72. August Hirsch, *Biographisches Lexikon der hervorragenden Ärzte aller Zeiten*, 2nd ed. (Berlin: Urban & Schwarzenberg), vol. 4 (1932) and vol. 1 (1929).

3

The Contribution of Exiled Portuguese Jews in Renaissance Medical Ethics

The aftermath of the edict of 1492 (which forced Muslims and Jews of Spain unwilling to convert into exile) continued to supply news items in Europe into the seventeenth century. Especially after Portugal was annexed to Spain by Philip II in 1580, there were waves of forced conversions and emigrations. The *Mercure français*, a publication close to what we would call a news magazine, summarized for its readers of 1613 a bit of Spanish history to serve as background to the events of 1610, i.e. renewed movements of refugees after Philip III enforced a new version of the old edict. (The new version expelled also "New Christians.") In the same publication, the motives for the original edict are given as two rather conflicting and thus ambiguous ones: good zeal (*bon zèle*) and the desire to confiscate the wealth of Jews and Moors in Spain. Then the magazine adds an equally ambiguous analysis of the original edict's consequences:

> And some have even said the Ordinance had been nice in appearance but of dangerous consequence; because the 100,000 Jews who did not want to obey it went to the country of the Turk, bringing with them the invention of cannons and of powder; those who had themselves baptized have since allied themselves with the noble families of Spain, contaminating them with their blood and belief.[1]

We learn in the same publication that Henri IV decreed (22 Feb. 1610) that the Christianized Jews could stay in France, but that the others had to leave. (He ordered the rich to pay the fare for the poor.) Several years later (i.e. in 1617, recording events of 1615), the *Mercure français* reports a rumor that Jews from Portugal intend to come from Holland to France and mentions a *commandement* banning all Jews. We are told that some Jews were surprised in Paris at a pascal meal

49

. . . and that they were ordered to leave the kingdom, in spite of the favors that Philoteus Elianus Montalto, a Portuguese physician with a high reputation at court, can procure them. This Montalto was of Jewish origin (*estoit Juif de race*): he died at Tours at the end of that year [1615]. His writings can be found in print.[2]

Such news clips from the early seventeenth century (of which the last grudgingly recognizes the role played by a distinguished physician in supporting his coreligionists) are only background for my topic, the contribution of some exiled Portuguese Jews in Renaissance medical ethics. 1614 is the date of publication of Rodrigo a Castro's *Medicus-Politicus*, possibly a milestone in the history of medical ethics, fully deserving the prominence I will give it in this chapter. In starting with the contemporary accounts of a serial publication, I would like to cut through hundreds of years of obfuscating scholarship and to discuss contemporary (sixteenth- to seventeenth-century) attitudes to Jewish physicians. Not that I pursue the illusionary aim of establishing *wie es wirklich gewesen* (to use Ranke's celebrated dictum); but my problem in this chapter is partly historiographic: there is a tradition of concealing the Jewishness of the émigré Portuguese physicians, like that of many other Iberians, out of national pride or religious prejudice. Relying on original publications and on the work of such scholars as Friedenwald, Jonathan Israel, Yerushalmi, Zagorin, Ruderman, and Hsia, I intend to take the Jewishness of the Portuguese physicians seriously: it is part of my subject.

Since, as we saw, Castro was possibly the first to problematize medical deception in an important way, we will set the issue of justifying pretense and lying in the context of the particular Marrano and New Christian experience by adducing the disquisition on lying by another Portuguese physician, writing in Spain; then we will consider the reputation of Jewish physicians as discussed in some Spanish medical works of the period and select one topic from a work in defense of Jewish doctors (by an Italian physician) for comparison with Castro's treatment, namely the controversy over whether physicians could refuse to treat their enemies. This "contextualizing" will be rounded off by a discussion of Protestant attacks against Castro (and against Jewish physicians in general) and of some works by Roman Catholic physicians writing in the genre of which the *Medicus-Politicus* is the finest Renaissance example.

Lusitani *Physicians and the Problem of Lying*

As we saw in the previous chapter, possibly the most ingenious stories of curing the imagination by imagination, that is, of curing it by pretense, are by Abraham Zacuto (or Zacutus Lusitanus, 1575–1642), who in his voluminous works shows an abiding interest in medical ethics and its history. Zacuto, grandson of his even more famous namesake, the astrologer driven from Castille to Portugal in the second half of the fifteenth century, was born in Lisbon to Christian parents of Jewish origin. After studying in Salamanca and Coimbra and receiving the medical doctorate at Siguenza when he was about twenty years old, he practiced in Lisbon for thirty years. At the age of fifty, he had to leave because, as Zedler's old encyclopedia puts it not only pointedly but inaccurately, "he turned to the superstition of his parents." According to the early biographies quoted by Friedenwald, he left "because a most cruel edict of the king of Lusitania banished all of the Hebrew stock from the kingdom."[3] Zacutus went to the Netherlands (Amsterdam and The Hague), where he joined the Jewish community and continued to practice medicine while writing his voluminous works, including the one on which his reputation is mainly based, *De medicorum principum historia.*

Like Abraham Zacutus, Rodrigo a Castro (1564–1627) identifies himself as "Lusitanus" in all his publications, and also like Zacutus, is imbued with the medicine of Spain, where he received his medical training. Complimentary letters exchanged and printed in their respective publications (including those of Rodrigo's son Benedict) attest to their relationship of mutual respect. Rodrigo a Castro came to Hamburg about 1594 as a prominent member of the important group of Lusitani that settled there at that time. In fact his son Jacob was the first child born to this group of Jews (most of them merchants) after it had gained formal recognition through a contract with the Hamburg senate.[4] Quite often Castro's references and examples are explicitly Spanish or Portuguese, though intended for an audience that is not: for instance, he holds up Spanish medical education as a model, refers to diagnosing some Spanish sailors in 1588 (the year of the Armada) who, "sick of the sea or of the war," pretended to be genuinely ill; reports that "in all of Spain" music is used (medically) to reestablish a balance of the humors; or describes the post-partum depression of a noble Portuguese lady (possibly one of the earliest and most articulate indentifications of this condition).[5]

Other than occasional references to detractors, very little is known about the difficulties Castro or Zacuto faced in either their old or their new countries. Harry Friedenwald wrote that "there is a curious absence of information concerning Zacutus's life in Lisbon" (p. 310). To what compromises and pretenses had he to subject himself to lead a professional life in Lisbon for thirty years? Similarly, we know nothing about the dilemma in which Castro must have seen himself before and after Philip II renewed the strict enforcement of laws against Jews. Possibly the group of well-educated Portuguese with which he came to Hamburg was looked upon as consisting of crypto-Catholics rather than crypto-Jews, although pretty soon after its arrival the truth must have become apparent. Why, one wonders, did Castro purchase a lot in the Catholic cemetery there?[6] Some distinguished recent scholarship on the plight of Spanish and Portuguese Jews, New Christians, and Marranos (particularly by Yerushalmi and Zagorin) has given an impressive picture of life on the Iberian peninsula amid persecution and intimidation.[7] Zagorin has linked the daily compromises Marranos were obliged to make to more general discussions of truth and falsehood in the period. (As he explains, *marrano* meant "pig" or "unclean," which led to its later meaning of a Jew pretending to be a Christian while secretly adhering to Judaism [p. 40].) In the picture that emerges, only secrecy assured survival, as family members informed on other family members and testified before the Inquisition (Zagorin, p. 56). When, for instance, was it safe to initiate a child into the Jewish faith? The physician Isaac Orobio de Castro (possibly a distant relative of Rodrigo's), convicted by the Inquisition *in absentia* and burned in effigy after escaping to Amsterdam, notes that "the greatest danger to Marranos comes from the children, and that therefore the parents divulge such information to them only at the age of twenty."[8] After the edict of 1492, there are reports of Marrano families going to the homes of other families for celebrating the sabbath with the women carrying spindles and distaffs to disguise their intent to their neighbors (Zagorin, p. 52). The emotionally charged atmosphere of the Counter-Reformation affected not only the Iberian peninsula but all countries under papal influence, as David Rudermann has shown in his studies of Jewish physicians in Italy, especially of Abraham Yagel; for legislation imposed by Pope Paul IV (1476–1559) and his successors led to increased impoverishment, ghettoization, and expulsion of Jews.[9]

The plight of the Marranos was to dissimulate, although, as Zagorin points out, they were "nevertheless not justly guilty of betraying the Christian faith, since it was a religion in which they had no belief" (p. 52). But to use the distinction we saw pointed out in Theodor Zwinger's *Theatrum vitae humanae* between dissimulation and simulation, if one follows Zagorin's justification (presumably their own) of *simulatio*, i.e. their pretending to be Christians, was this not different from their *dissimulatio*, concealing their beliefs? Although Zagorin does not distinguish the terms "simulation" and "dissimulation," for my purposes he asks the central question: "Orobio de Castro also declared that it was impossible to live in Spain without dissimulation. But how then did Marranos defend their dissembling and double life?" (p. 56). The answer he gives is not simple, and I can summarize only some of the highlights.

As in Protestantism, where there is a difference between the complying "Nicodemists" and the rigorous and intransigent "anti-Nicodemists" of Calvin's persuasion, there are at least two traditions also in Judaism. Complying and dissimulating Marranos could find solace in Maimonides's thoughts on forced conversion. While Maimonides had the highest admiration for those willing to be martyrs, the gist of his letter on the subject was "a compassionate concern for the many who were incapable of such heroism" (Zagorin, p. 57). But on the other side, Zagorin points out, "Isaac Caro, a Castillian rabbi who left Spain in 1492, rejected Maimonides's arguments exonerating the convert who yielded to compulsion" (p. 60). After discussing various modes of crypto-Jews' defenses of their existence, Zagorin points to the similarity of their rationale to that of the Protestants under Catholic princes in England and suppressed Catholics under Queen Elizabeth and King James, and has to concede that doctrines justifying pretended and deceitful conformity emerged in all these places and that these doctrines have parallel features: "The theory and practice of dissimulation as we have seen it in the case of crypto-Judaism were never a peculiarity of any single religious body. They were the inevitable consequence of Christian religious oppression against Jews and Christians alike, as well as a common product of a religious tradition based on the scriptures" (pp. 61–62).

It would be foolish indeed to expect that physicians of Jewish origin from the Iberian peninsula would subscribe to one and the same view about deception, and particularly medical deception.

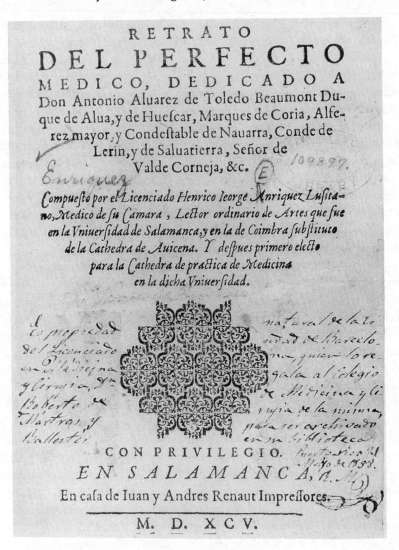

RETRATO
DEL PERFECTO
MEDICO, DEDICADO A
Don Antonio Aluarez de Toledo Beaumont Duque de Alua, y de Huefcar, Marques de Coria, Alferez mayor, y Condeftable de Nauarra, Conde de Lerin, y de Saluatierra, Señor de Valde Corneja, &c.

Compuefto por el Licenciado Henrico Ieorge Anriquez Lufitano, Medico de fu Camara, Lector ordinario de Artes que fue en la Vniuerfidad de Salamanca, y en la de Coimbra fubftituto de la Cathedra de Auicena. Y defpues primero electo para la Cathedra de practica de Medicina en la dicha Vniuerfidad.

CON PRIVILEGIO.
EN SALAMANCA,
En cafa de Iuan y Andres Renaut Impreffores.

M. D. XCV.

Figure 3.1. Frontispiece of Henrique Jorge Henriques, *Retrato del perfecto médico*, Madrid, 1595 (National Library of Medicine).

However, the Marrano world of Portugal that Rodrigo a Castro escaped may have made him especially sensitive to the truth-versus-falsehood issues he discusses with greater clarity than any other physician of his period, in the chapter entitled, "Whether the physician may legitimately lie in the interest of cure." While particularly sensitive to moral questions of this kind, he would, in his predicament, naturally have tended to justify the use of ruses also in medicine.

We may follow up this matter by a limited counterproof. One of the predecessors of Castro's *Medicus-Politicus* was the *Retrato del perfecto médico* (1595), by Henrique Jorge Henriques (or Enriquez or Anriquez). Although more modest in its intellectual aspirations and less rigorous (and more anecdotal) in its construction, this dialogue between a theologian and a physician is in some ways the closest ancestor to Castro's work. But if I have found no proof that Castro used it, this may be because Castro was trying to give the impression that his project (to write about the *oeconomia* and *politia* of medicine) was a novel affair, although he qualified his claim sufficiently to acknowledge the potential existence of works like Henriques' *Portrait of the Perfect Physician*: he called his own undertaking so exceptional (*egregium*) that "scarcely anyone has yet dared to attempt it."[10] Lope de Vega wrote two sonnets to Henriques, and in the nineteenth century, the medical historian Antonio Hernández Morejón praised Henriques' book to the sky.[11] Henriques, who calls himself "Lusitanus" on the title page, came from the town of Guarda in the Province of Beyra (Portugal) and studied at Salamanca under the famous physicians Tomás Rodriguez da Veiga and Ambrosio Nuñez, both "Lusitani" and of Jewish descent. The works of both of these, incidentally, will be singled out by Rodrigo a Castro and recommended for the library of his ideal physician.[12] One of Lope de Vega's sonnets on Henriques claims, in an elegant compliment, that the model for the *Retrato del perfecto médico* was Henriques himself.[13] But since Lope de Vega, despite anti-Jewish sentiment in his plays, had good relations with New Christians and even Marranos, his high esteem for the physician proves nothing about the latter's background.

I have no evidence that Henriques was a New Christian or of Jewish descent, except for the bare facts just mentioned plus a few conjectures. Yerushalmi has observed that the incursion into Spain of Portuguese New Christians was of such dimension and impact that, to the Spaniards of the seventeenth century, 'Portuguese' was virtually synonymous with 'Jew' (p. 10). As we shall see later, this holds true not only for Spain, for "Lusitanus" became a continuing self-identification for Rodrigo a Castro's physician son Benedict, who called himself by that epithet in his publications although he was born in Hamburg. Since Henriques obtained a chair of philosophy at

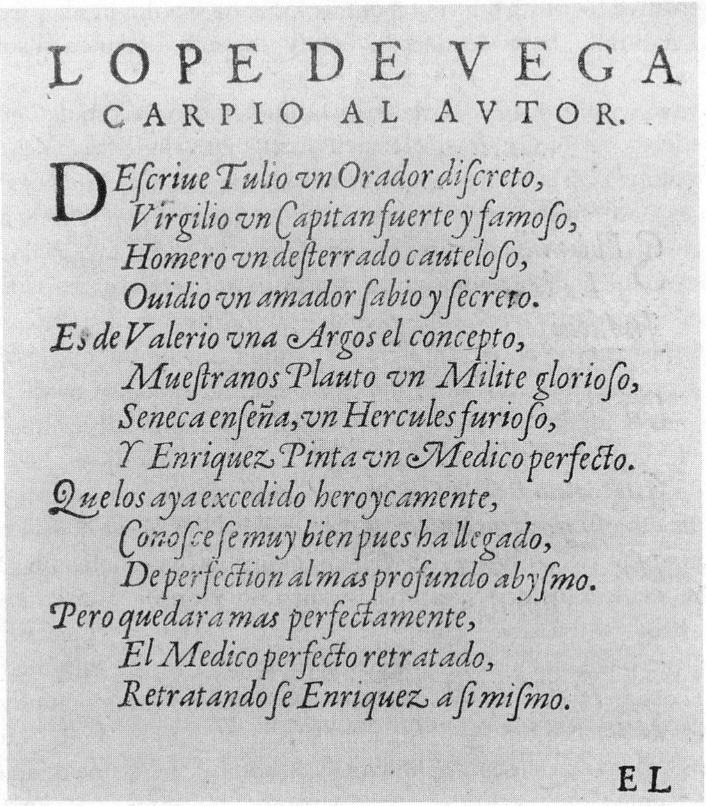

LOPE DE VEGA
CARPIO AL AVTOR.

DEfcriue Tulio vn Orador difcreto,
    Virgilio vn Capitan fuerte y famofo,
Homero vn defterrado cautelofo,
Ouidio vn amador fabio y fecreto.
Es de Valerio vna Argos el concepto,
    Mueftranos Plauto vn Milite gloriofo,
Seneca enfeña, vn Hercules furiofo,
    Y Enriquez Pinta vn Medico perfecto.
Que los aya excedido heroycamente,
    Conofce fe muy bien pues ha llegado,
De perfection al mas profundo abyfmo.
Pero quedara mas perfectamente,
    El Medico perfecto retratado,
Retratandofe Enriquez a fi mifmo.

EL

Figure 3.2. Poem by Lope de Vega in Henriques, *Retrato del perfecto médico*, Madrid, 1595, Sig. tt^v (National Library of Medicine).

Salamanca and then a chair of medicine at Coimbra, his credentials, if he was a New Christian, would have had to be quite extraordinary.

The "perfect physician" delineated by Henriques of course fulfills the duties officially mandated by the Church (making sure, for instance, that the sacraments are administered to the gravely ill), but the book also demonstrates caution about possible censorship. Thus, on the page on which Henriques recommends that the perfect physician should be married, since, as he puts it, the union of two bodies and two minds yields the greatest contentment, he adds a palinode (in Latin) in the margin: happier and more tranquil still is celibate life![14]

When the subject of lying comes up in this work, the phrase "the Lord our God very much abhors the lie" (pp. 252–53) sets the tone.

Even before that, when in the discussion of what kind of sport or relaxation might be seemly for the ideal physician Henriques finds games (presumably cards and dice) unsuitable—since *mentira*, lying, is connected with them—one senses something like a puritan rigor. He quotes Ambrose's statement that "all those who love the untruth are sons of the devil" (p. 256), and the very passage from Aristotle (according to which lying is an evil in and of itself) that Castro will oppose to Plato and the medical tradition. But in contrast to Castro's later discussion, Henriques presents no moral dilemma nor problem of ethics, nor does the issue ever turn specifically medical.

Curiously, whatever doubts there may be about the need to lie, for Henriques the Naaman story (4 Reg. 5 or 2 Kings 5) clinches the issue—he retells it in considerable detail. It is the story of the Syrian military captain Naaman, a leper, who is sent by his own king to the king of Israel in the hope of finding a cure for his disease. After being cured (somewhat against his expectations) merely by dipping several times into the Jordan at the prophet Elisha's behest, he offers Elisha rich gifts to express his gratitude, all of which the prophet refuses to accept. However, after Naaman has departed, Elisha's servant Gehazi runs after him, pretending to Naaman that Elisha has changed his mind. When his ruse is discovered, Gehazi is punished with Naaman's skin disease ("leprosy")—a moral example of how much God detests lying.

Henriques drives home this point so singlemindedly that in the process he omits the two verses in the story that would have had considerable resonance for conversos: the healed and converted Naaman worries that in Syria he will be obliged to appear worshiping the false gods of his lord. He says to Elisha: "In this thing the Lord pardon thy servant, that when my master goeth to worship there, and he leaneth on my hand, and I bow myself in the house of Rimmon: when I bow myself in the house of Rimmon, the Lord pardon thy servant in this thing. And he [Elisha] said unto him [Naaman], Go in peace" (2 Kings 5:18–19). In fact, while the story of Naaman at the most obvious level contrasts justified pretense (Naaman in the temple) with detestable ruses (Gehazi), Henriques, to support his rigorist position, presents only the latter.

Henriques' selection of one side of the biblical story is not trivial and cannot be accidental. As Zagorin has pointed out, Elisha's response to Naaman was one of the main texts, possibly *the* text justifying dissimulation, ever since the learned medieval exegete Nicholas

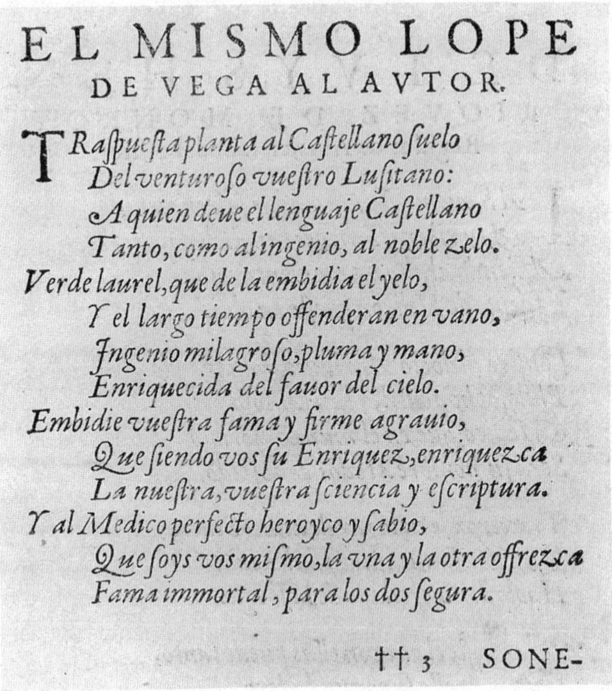

EL MISMO LOPE
DE VEGA AL AVTOR.

TRaſpueſta planta al Caſtellano ſuelo
  Del venturoſo vueſtro Luſitano:
A quien deue el lenguaje Caſtellano
Tanto, como al ingenio, al noble zelo.
Verde laurel, que de la embidia el yelo,
  Y el largo tiempo offenderan en vano,
  Ingenio milagroſo, pluma y mano,
  Enriquecida del fauor del cielo.
Embidie vueſtra fama y firme agrauio,
  Que ſiendo vos ſu Enriquez, enriquezca
  La nueſtra, vueſtra ſciencia y eſcriptura.
Y al Medico perfecto heroyco y ſabio,
  Que ſoys vos miſmo, la vna y la otra offrezca
  Fama immortal, para los dos ſegura.

††3   SONE-

Figure 3.3.   Poem by Lope de Vega in Henriques, *Retrato del perfecto médico*, Madrid, 1595, Sig. tt3 (National Library of Medicine).

of Lyra had meticulously analyzed the passage. This is Zagorin's summary of Nicholas's analysis of Elisha's response to Naaman:

> According to Nicholas [of Lyra], the prophet told Naaman that the action he feard as unlawful was lawful. Naaman had a duty to assist his king, and this was not illicit in its own nature. Moreover, he could perform his duty whether outside or within the idol's temple, just as a Christian girl captured by the Saracens may carry her mistress's train into a Muslim temple without worshiping Muhammed. What Naaman asked of Elisha, therefore, was that he might perform the same duty to his master in the idol's temple as he lawfully did elsewhere. He sought this permission not from reverence to the idol but lest he incur the king's displeasure. This was what Elisha granted him, Nicholas concludes, and it was not unlawful.[15]

Given the fact that Nicholas of Lyra would have been part of any worthwhile biblical commentary and in the presence of dozens of Renaissance references to the story of Naaman as a document legitimizing a certain kind of outward behavior,[16] it seems impossible that the *catedrático de filosofía* at the famous University of Salamanca and later holder of the Avicenna chair at Coimbra would have been unfamiliar with such contexts. While it is rarely safe to build an argument on the absence of an element, in this case Henriques' retelling of the story of Naaman without those crucial verses, that is, his wrenching it out of its ordinary frame of reference and merely making the point that liars may incur leprosy by God's wrath, gives his disquisition on falsehood an extraordinary edge or even shrillness.

The contrast with the way Rodrigo a Castro presents the question whether falsehood can be justified (in a book of essentially the same genre) could not be greater. As we saw in the last chapter, Castro unfolds the problem as a controversy between Plato and Aristotle. Plato (according to a quotation from the *Republic*) appears to justify falsehood as a remedy or form of medicine (*pharmakon*) useful to the physicians, but not to the laymen (*idiotai*).[17] The ancient physicians Castro adduces demonstrate the necessity of occasional deception. But then, according to Castro, "Aristotle fights on the other side" (p. 143) for—as Henriques knew—in his *Nicomachean Ethics* he praises truthfulness in itself, even when nothing depends on it (bk. 4, chap. 5). We have already noted how Castro resolves the "controversy" with the help of the casuistic distinction between a harmful and a helpful or officious lie (*mendacium nocivum* and *mendacium officiosum*), likening the officious lie to hellebore which, administered without discrimination, is deadly, but in certain situations can be wholesome. Aristotle, he claims, had in mind only useless or harmful lies.

After minimally outlining the Marrano context of dissimulation and also Henriques' rigorist disquisition on the topic in the same context as Castro's, namely for delineating the ideal physician, we will find it more difficult to dismiss Castro's discussion as a mere display of clever philosophizing through adjusting conflicting authorities. Most important, Castro's solution will strike one as balanced, humane, and possibly urbane. At the margin of what is demonstrable, I would further suggest that Castro's use of the Platonic passage with its hierarchical imperative is not so innocent. Plato seems to assume that a falsehood as a *pharmakon* is uncontroverted, since the point he is leading up to is that "rulers of the city may if anybody, fitly lie on

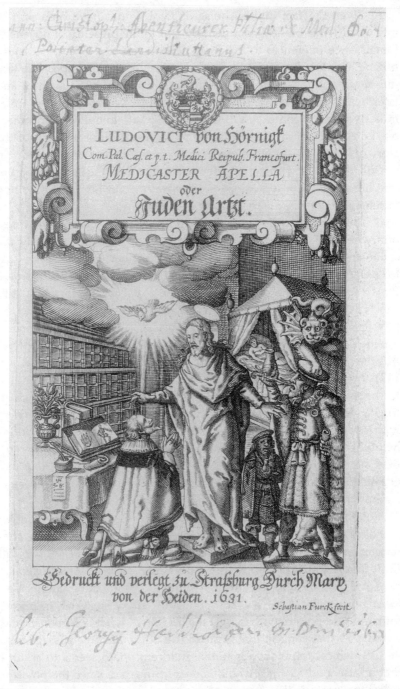

Figure 3.4. Fontispiece of Ludwig von Hörnigk, *Medicaster Apella*, Strassburg, 1631 (National Library of Medicine).

account of enemies or citizens for the benefit of state." This notion had an extraordinary fortune, as is shown, for instance, in Bacon's essay on dissimulation, which restricts everyone except kings and princes to telling the truth. Of course, we should guard against a modern misreading of Castro's title *Medicus-Politicus* as doctor-politician: as we saw earlier, Castro's subject includes the part of the physician's activity covered by the words *oeconomia* and *politia*, i.e. how to adjust the patients' environment to the conditions of their cure (rather than how to diagnose and treat specific diseases); and von Hörnigk's *Politia medica* (1638) seems to have imitated that usage.[18] But in writing a work that he dedicated to the Hamburg senate, Castro may indeed be implying something of what a modern reader senses here: he may be inverting the direction of the analogy and arguing from the assumed or known ruler:ruled relationship to the relationship of physician to patient that is to be explained. In that sense the title of the work, *Medicus-Politicus*, with its unusual if not ungrammatical hyphen, would be full of meaning.

However, before we can hope to come to grips with this problem and similar ones depending on context, we need to focus our attention on discussions of contemporary (i.e. sixteenth- and seventeenth-century) attitudes toward Jewish physicians, a task where some spadework is needed.

The Reputation of Jewish Physicians

A recent paper entitled "La renaissance et l'Ecole Iatroéthique Portugaise du XVIe siècle" (The Renaissance and the Portuguese School of Medical Ethics in the 16th century), the very subject I want to deal with here, speaks of the conception of an international and even "geopolitical" flow of ideas on the entire planet during the Renaissance, as exemplified by the close contacts between the universities of Salamanca and Bologna and by the string of eminent Portuguese physicians, formed at Salamanca, spreading to all parts of Europe. The phenomenon is interpreted as part of "a group of new basic ideas conceived through the Discoveries and spread by Portuguese humanism through Europe, and from the end of the sixteenth century consolidated in the union with Spain of that period."[19] Among the seven physicians whose works are highlighted are Pedro Nuñes, Amatus Lusitanus, Tomás Rodrigues da Veiga, Rodrigo a Castro, and Abraham Zacuto, all of whom either came from Jewish families (and were New

Christians or Marranos) or professed Judaism. In addition, the author discusses the work of Henriques, about whose origins we cannot be sure, but about whom I expressed some conjectures in the previous section. But oddly enough the paper never acknowledges the religious or racial tensions of the period—nor are the words *Jewish* or *Jew* used once. The closest the author comes to suggesting a particular motive for the spread of this "Portuguese humanism" is one sentence admitting obscurely and possibly in coded language that the Portuguese physicians did not leave for foreign parts attracted by university positions, but for other reasons: "Parallel [to these developments], there was an important medical emigration of Portuguese physicians to several countries of Europe, not for the sake of university teaching but in order to give assistance [as practical physicians], with even those aims permeated by ideas of the period and deeply imbued with Renaissance medical ideas."[20] The paper thus demonstrates for Renaissance Portugal an extreme version of the denial and neglect of Jewish origins that Stephen Gilman has observed in scholarship on authors from Renaissance Spain. In his book on Fernando Rojas, author of *La Celestina*, Gilman writes: "The Jewish origins of many Spaniards of the past are first denied (in the case of Rojas, as recently as 1967); and then, if the denial cannot stand up in the face of the evidence, they are ignored."[21]

The difficult and sometimes embattled position of Jews in the Renaissance is evident from the period's apologias or defenses of Judaism, which are divided (by Yerushalmi) into two kinds: apologetic works defending Judaism or explaining it to the Gentiles; and active polemics assailing Christianity, for obvious reasons in manuscript. For the limited subject of medicine, that is, apologias of Jewish physicians, I know only two works entirely devoted to such defense: the books by David de Pomis and Benedict a Castro (son of Rodrigo), both of which will concern us later.[22] Of course the defenses by De Pomis and a Castro would belong in Yerushalmi's first category. There are, however, other treatments defending Jewish physicians, more incidental and even indirect, perhaps, but not any less important, and written in full awareness of a string of papal pronouncements against Jews in medicine. I find such accounts in Spain, of all countries, at the time of the renewed effort to expel not only Jews but also converts, for fear that they might be Marranos.

In discussing the question whether Egypt is the region most suitable for developing the imagination (declared by him an essential faculty for developing all branches of science), the sixteenth-century physician Juan Huarte de San Juan says that ultimately it is the excellence of Jewish physicians that makes him lean toward the praise of Egypt. I am quoting from an Elizabethan translation of Huarte's *Examen de ingenios*:

> But the argument which most over-ruleth me in this behalfe, is, that when *Francis* of *Valois* king of France, was molested by a long infirmitie, and saw that the Phisitians of his houshold and court, could yeeld him no remedy, he would say every time when his fever increased, It was not possible that any Christian Phisition could cure him, neither at their hands did he ever hope for recoverie: wherethrough one time agreeved to see himselfe thus vexed with his fever, he dispatched a post into Spaine, praieng the emperour *Charles* the fifth, that he would send him a Jew Phisition, the best of his court, touching whom he had understood, that he was able to yeeld him remedie for his sicknesse, if by art it might be effected. At this request the Spaniards made much game, and all of them concluded it was an humorous conceit of a man, whose brains were turmoiled with the fever. But for all this, the Emperour gave commandement that such a Phisition should be sought out, if anie there were, though to find him they should be driven to send out of his dominions; and when none could be met withall, he sent a Phisition newly made a Christian, supposing that he might serve to satisfie the kings humour. But the Phisition being arrived in France, and brought to the kings presence; there passed between them a gratious discourse, in which it appeared that the Phisition was a Christian: and therefore the king would receive no phisicke at his hands. The king with opinion which he had conceived of the phisition, that he was an Hebrue, by way of passing the time, asked him whether he were not as yet weary in looking for the Messias promised in the law? The phisition answered; Sir I expect not any Messias promised in the Jews law. You are verie wise in that (replied the king): for the tokens which were delivered in the divine scripture, whereby to know his comming, are all fulfilled manie daies ago. This number of daies (reioyned the phisition) we Christians do well reckon: for there are now finished 1542 yeares; in the end of which he died on the crosse, and the third day rose again, and afterwards ascended into heaven,

where he now remaineth. Why then quoth the king you are a Christian? yea, Sir, by the grace of God, I am a Christian (quoth the phisition) then (answered the king) return you home to your own dwelling in good time: for in mine owne house and court I have Christian phisitions very excellent, and I held you for a Jew, who (in mine opinion) are those that have best natu-rall abilitie to cure my disease. After this maner he licenced him without once suffering him to feele his pulse, or see his state, or telling him one word of his griefe. And forthwith he sent to Con-stantinople for a Jew, who healed him with onely milke of the she Asse.[23]

Even shaped as the anecdote is to make a particular point, one senses the double-bind in which the physician of Jewish origin was placed. First, in order to be close to the Spanish king's court and generally to avoid prosecution in Spain, he had to be a Christian. Therefore, and also given the papal bulls against Jewish physicians (from Pope Paul IV [1555] to Gregory XIII [1581]), it is reasonable for him to expect, once he arrives at the French court, that similar rules obtain there and that a profession of Christian faith is demanded—ironically this expec-tation is not fulfilled.

Huarte's assent to the notion of Jewish superiority in medicine, first suggested indirectly, soon becomes entirely unambiguous. Described through bemused Spanish reaction to the fancy of a fever-ish brain, the French king's idea soon becomes a major theme of his book, namely the insight sometimes available in certain conditions of distemperedness. This is how Huarte commits himself: "This imagina-tion of king *Francis* (as I think) was verie true, and I have so con-ceived it to be, for that in the great hot distemperatures of the brain, I have proved tofore, how the imagination findeth out that, which (the partie being sound) could never have done" (p. 185). Indeed, Huarte insists another time that "it shall not seem that I have spoken in jest." His view is, moreover, supported by his firm beliefs about operative links between region/climate/diet on the one hand and the human mind on the other (most notably the imagination), notions ultimately derived but transmuted from classical medicine, in which the influ-ence of climate and region are *causae non naturales*. (In the nineteenth century, ideas about blood and soil would lead, with respect to the Jews, to opposite results). Thus, according to Huarte, people living in the region of Spain are not particularly gifted in medicine because of their want of imagination; nor, certainly, are those peoples further north, since their imagination is very slow and slack, only suited "to make clocks, pictures, poppets, and other ribaldries which are impertinent for mans service" (p. 183). In addition to the influence of region (Egypt), he speculates at length about the role of the manna that sustained the tribe of Israel in the desert, specifically whether its effect could continue in the descendants of those who tasted of it: "There presenteth itself a difficultie verie great against all these things reherced by us, and that is, that if the children or nephews of those who were in Aegypt and enjoyed the Manna, the water and the subtle air of the wildernesse, had been made choice of for phisitions, it might seeme, that king *Francis* opinion were in some part probable, for the reasons by us reported" (p. 194)—but would not those influences be lost by now, centuries later? He finally resolves the issue by declaring that the special disposition of that seed would take three thousand years to be entirely obliterated (p. 196).

Huarte's admiration for Jewish physicians has not gone unnoticed. On the basis of it and of some other characteristics of his work, Malcom K. Reed has surmised that Huarte himself was a converso. Drawing on Stephen Gilman's work for support, he writes: "Huarte's obsessive concern to exclude religious considerations from his scientific investigation reminds us that the *converso* was typically skeptical and irreligious, committed above all to a rationalistic view of life. Though not agnostic in the modern sense of these terms, the *converso* forced to abandon his own religion and unable to embrace sincerely that of his oppressors, sometimes surrendered to doubt and uncertainty."[24] Reed also points out that the practitioners of the black arts were traditionally of Jewish descent. Therefore Huarte, in his attempt to rationalize magic and insanity (according to Reed), captures perfectly the converso yearning to explain and control the supernatural. Reed further surmises that "perhaps it was the insecurity of his marginal status in society that led Huarte, like many *conversos*, to seek a basis for personal evaluation in such superficial criteria as honor, rank and dress." Finally he even inverts Huarte's insistence (in his name) that he hailed from the Basque country (thus by implication claiming descent from Old Christians) and reads that as another indication that he was a converso.

I admit that I feel progressively uneasy as I go down that list of arguments. Even the first, that conversos are typically irreligious and skeptical, is useful only as a general reminder and can hardly serve as a criterion for identifying conversos. Insistence on the physician's cleanliness and neatness of dress (if that is intended) is a commonplace in medical literature since antiquity. Finally, the argument from the name (or place name) at most exemplifies the no-win situation the candidate might have faced at the time of the Inquisition, but beyond that does not carry much conviction.

More interesting is the claim that Jewish physicians excel all others because of the Egyptian experience of the tribe of Israel, and also the manner it which it is presented. That Huarte insists he is not jesting indicates that he is not merely repeating a received idea or something self-evident in a country where, in the Middle Ages, the majority of physicians had been Jewish.[25] In the Spain of Huarte's time, his insistence would have taken a considerable amount of courage. Most significantly, the claim of Jewish excellence in medicine is repeated in the *Retrato del perfecto médico* by Henriques, a physician whom one could more defensibly consider a New Christian, since he identified himself as "Lusitanus," a term which (as we saw earlier), with the wave of immigration from Portugal about that time, begins to indicate more than mere geographic origin.

Henriques gets to the subject with a reference to Galen, according to whom the proper appellation of the physician should be *inventor occasioni* (the inventor for an occasion). He then refers to "the subtle Doctor Huarte" according to whom the *ingenio* (mind, genius) of the Egyptians "or of those whose ancestors lived in Egypt, as those deriving from the Hebrews" is most apt for medicine. Then he—or rather his theologian Arcediano—tells the anecdote of King Francis writing to Charles V requesting a Jewish physician from his court, the laughter at the Spanish court, and the sending of "un Medico Christiano nuevo" (p. 145). After the French king's seeming whim and his cure by a properly Jewish physician from Constantinople have been reported, Henriques has his *licenciado*, the medical partner in the imagined dialogue, give the "scientific" explanation (from humoral physiology) of the French king's insight while seriously ill: a certain moderate warmth enhances imaginative powers. The *licenciado* quotes at length from the relevant text, pseudo-Aristotle's *Problem XXX, 1*, including the passage about the Syracusan poet whose work was more distinguished when he was out of his mind.[26] Since the ancient sybils are also mentioned in that passage, Henriques' spokesman is careful to note that the Catholic Church allows for the possibility that in their prophecies the sybils were divinely inspired (without, however, mentioning the Christian commonplace that all such oracles fell silent at the birth of Christ): ". . . since for so high a matter natural genius, however sudden, did not suffice."[27] While the comment seems partly motivated by Henriques' fear of laying himself open to charges of naturalistic-humoral explanation of divine prophecy, it also has the effect of associating the French king's conception of Jewish physicians with prophetic and even divine insight.

In substance, Henriques' retelling of the anecdote in the form of a dialogue adds little to it: the passage on melancholic insight (from pseudo-Aristotle) is extremely well known in the Renaissance and of course adduced in Huarte's *Examen de ingenios* in similar contexts. As in many works of the period, the dialogue form he creates in imitation of Cicero and other ancient models is only a didactic device, in fact a pseudodialogue. As with the issue of whether the perfect physician is married or celibate, mentioned earlier, the "real" dialogue happens between the text recounting the justification for the French king's preference and the comment in the margin. While the text is in Castilian, the margin says in Latin: "Because of the nobility of medicine, Augustinus of Ancona in his *De potestate ecclesiastica* and Antoninus of Florence in his *Summa* pars 3, tit. 7, c. 2 said that *spurii* [those of uncertain origin, those who do not know their father or mother] should not be admitted to medicine because they are not worthy of such high nobility."[28] At the place indicated, Antoninus says (with reference to Augustinus of Ancona) that physicians are not to be admitted to the practice of medicine unless they are sworn in and "derive from a legitimate marriage."[29] Does Henriques want to suggest by his marginal note that only the Jewish physicians are of legitimate ancestry (since they are closer to the Egyptian experience of Israel)—a true, rather than the accepted *hidalgía* and real *limpieza*? Of course this would be a deliberate misreading of the *summistae*, who are very precise in their language and do not use the word *spurii* in this context. Or was Henriques covering his flank by intimating that he was not including in his praise of Jewish physicians just any quack of uncertain ancestry (particularly if Malcolm Reed is correct in his view that "the practitioners of the black arts were traditionally of Jewish stock"[30])? In any case, for Henriques, a "Lusitanus" (which, as we saw, may mean more than just "Portuguese"), to invoke the notion of legitimate ancestry in a margin facing the argument for the excellence of Jewish physicians would seem to be a daring move, a serious game perhaps, accentuated further and ironically by the fact that the summist's chapter referred to is the very one (in fact the very page and even column) spelling out the prohibition against seeking help from Jewish physicians except in an emergency and laying out the punishments for infraction: demotion for a cleric (*deponatur*) and excommunication for lay people.

It was while laboring under such prohibitions in Italy (the bull by Gregory XIII was published 1585) that the physician and practicing rabbi David de Pomis (1525–1600) wrote his apology for Jewish physicians, *De medico hebraeo enarratio apologetica* (1588). De Pomis does not recount the French king's preference for a Jewish physician, but urges the reader (*obsecro*) to read an account by the French king's geographer of the preeminence of Jewish physicians in Turkey.[31] August Hirsch's biographical dictionary acknowledges that David de Pomis led a migratory life, persecuted by individual bishops, but neither Hirsch nor Harry Friedenwald, who translates portions of section 11 of the defense (with its reference to his "calumniators"), indicates the nature of the persecutions.[32] Thus we do not know what was "the abusive strife" (*contumeliosum certamen*) which, according to the opening of his dedication to the Duke of Urbino, prompted him to write this book. (He mentions incidentally that he had traveled to Turkey.) Although De Pomis obviously is not Portuguese, some of the issues he makes explicit are crucial to understanding Rodrigo a Castro, who leaves them implicit. De Pomis's *Enarratio apologetica* necessarily represents the first of Yerushalmi's two types of apologias: it is addressed to the Christian reader, and always temperate, balanced, and urbane.

According to De Pomis, the proper physician naturally professes religion or professes a natural religion, since he has constant proof from all living beings and "the texture of our body" (*corporis fabrica*, p. 6)—the words have a Vesalian ring—that God exists; hence the physician follows and venerates God with a "natural love" (*naturali amore*). Thus any physician ought to be "the servant of Divine Majesty" (p. 9). When Jewish physicians cure the poor, they do so out of compassion (*miseratio*), "which is in people naturally, as we just said."[33] For De Pomis, this "natural" compassion is part of the meaning of *humanitas*: "When we cure the lowly [or suppressed], this is an act of humanity, as we remind ourselves that all human beings are equally inserted in the chain of humanity."[34]

The point of the book is to demythologize the Christians' image of Jews and, more specifically, of the Jewish physician. De Pomis takes on a version of the rumor of ritual slaying of Christians by Jews, i.e. of what has been called the "blood libel," recently studied by Yerushalmi and (for Germany) by R. Po-Chia Hsia.[35] The libel comprises three accusations: homicide, the eating of blood, and the practice of magic arts. De Pomis argues against those who claim that Jewish physicians feel justified in killing their Christian patients or in detaining them from Christian rites (p. 10) and will return to these allegations in chapter 11 (of which we have Friedenwald's translation). He points out that such slander is contradicted by the "dogmas" of the Hippocratic oath, to which all physicians subscribe. This oath is like a "sacramental bond" (*vinculum sacramenti*), violation of which would be accounted "sacrilege" (p. 12).

The emphasis in this book is programmatically on the similarity between Christians and Jews. The charges of turpitude of Jewish physicians are so outrageous, De Pomis explains, because "Jew and Christian seem to differ little from another. . . . They worship one God and both affirm His wonderful deeds, which are the same. Both follow the same precepts, except for traditions and ceremonies. . . ."[36] Since this is so, "it can be clear even to the blind that the difference of religion between Jew and Christian is not so great as to make possible any such crime between them."[37] The author's words on friendship may have been far from commonplace then; in fact, in certain parts of the world they may sound revolutionary even now: "It is appropriate to say one thing about it in passing, namely that true friendship cannot be impeded in any way by time, age, or difference of religion."[38] After these strong words on the marriage of true minds, De Pomis confidently claims that it has yet to be demonstrated in his days that difference of religion can deflect a physician from doing his duty. He adds that by religious difference he means division among Christians, Turks, and Jews.

By quoting the wording of the prayer in question, De Pomis also disarms the allegation that Jews blaspheme Christians three times per day and pray for their destruction; the prayer mentions heretics, traitors, and "God's enemies," and none of these terms, he says, applies to Christians (p. 73). (Hsia has pointed out that Luther, among other sixteenth-century Germans, believed that Jews used black magic to harm Christians and practiced medicine to kill them,[39] and we will find these allegations repeated in the seventeenth century in Ludwig von Hörnigk's attack on Jewish physicians.) De Pomis argues at length (and will return to the subject in section 11) that Jews do not consider Christians or even Turks their enemies: "The surrounding nations, i.e. those inhabiting France, Germany, Spain, or even all of Europe are not truly our enemies, nor have ever been."[40] But since, as he reports, Christians wrongly assume that Jews hate Christians, he raises and answers the question how physicians, notably Jewish ones, behave toward their enemies. His answer is plain: the physician cures the rich and the poor, the high and the low, "enemies or those he specially cares for; and, again, those of his religion and those of a different one."[41]

Most interestingly, he describes the process by which the enemy, by seeking medical help from a physician of the opposing side, ceases to be an enemy and assumes the status of a captive or prisoner:

> If then we are duty-bound to give enemies medical assistance, we hold it for proven fact that we do not give them any less than proper medical care; and there is absolutely no ambiguity here: for since they have voluntarily delivered their lives into our hands, they are not our enemies anymore but rather straightway turn into our friends, whom to hurt in any manner is shameful, and who now are considered by us prisoners or vanquished.[42]

I cannot find in De Pomis any sign of "the more austere aspects of the ethos of rabbinic Judaism" that Yerushalmi claims Isaac Cardoso (the subject of his detailed study) absorbed a few decades later in Italy, and which Yerushalmi contrasts with the more humanistic concerns of Sephardic Jews. (Yerushalmi mentions De Pomis only in a footnote [p. 376].) It is true that De Pomis's aims may be considered narrowly apologetic and reactive, since he addresses himself only to misconceptions about Jewish physicians, his treatise being thus quite different from Cardoso's later *Excelencias de los Hebreos*. But for the history of medical ethics the work's emphasis on the bedrock of humanity that unites Christians, Jews, and Turks is important, as we shall consider more closely in connection with Rodrigo a Castro. At the same time, De Pomis adopts the language of the Christian by elevating the various elements of the oath attributed to the heathen Hippocrates to "dogmas" and even "sacraments."

Rodrigo a Castro's Medicus-Politicus: Not a Defense of Jewish Medicine

Herman Kellenbenz says somewhat cautiously about Castro's motivation for writing *Medicus-Politicus:* "Perhaps he [Castro] felt himself to be under attack not only as a physician, but also as a Jew, when in 1614 he published his treatise *Medicus-Politicus sive de Officiis medico-politicis Tractatus*. It is a kind of apology in which Castro expounds the duties of the physician and tried to prove the indispensability of medicine primarily with references to the Old Testament."[43] Although I do not think that the references to the Old Testament have the prominence claimed, I generally agree with the characterization if it is understood that the work is not an apology of or for the Jewish physician or even for Jewish medicine, but an apology for medicine by a Portuguese Jew in a specific predicament. These distinctions, which may seem excessively fine, in fact point to the work's aim: not to present an argument for Jewish, Christian, or Arabic medical ethics or medicine, but to present the duties of the physician as transcending these demarcations.

Although Castro sees himself as a "rational" (i.e. Galenic) physician and in defining medicine uses the phrase *medicina rationalis* (p. 4), he speaks for a humanistically liberal medical education, and in the context of specifying what a physician's library ought to contain, makes an argument for inclusion rather than exclusion: "Not that we cling so much to the authority of Galen alone that we may seem to be swearing by his words, as do those who despise all Arabs as barbaric. For philosophers and physicians ought to have freedom like the bees to choose whatever is best." While at the surface this is merely a plea for Arabic medicine, one might take it also for an indirect argument for Jewish medicine (not mentioned until the next clause, and in fact almost entirely absent from his book), for Castro goes on to say that what counts in the authors one selects is not whether they are Greek, Arab, Hebrew, or Latin, but whether they write the truth. But I hesitate to construe so much indirectness in an author who boldly speaks his mind on so many subjects. I prefer to stay with the surface sense which, on the basis of a distinction between medicine and religion, is that religious distinctions are not relevant to medicine and to judging medical authors. "For they [the medical authors] do not teach religion, but medicine. Plato is my friend, as is also Socrates; but a closer friend is truth."[44]

This is not an incidental comment; rather the Erasmian adage is a recurring and important theme for Castro, to which he returns a few pages later. Again he inveighs against those who by some whim or fancy reject Arabic physicians and condemn them by some "absurd vanity" (p. 95) together with the "barbarian" physicians, making exception only for Galen. This exception would seem to indicate that the "barbarians" are not medieval authors writing nonclassical Latin, but non-Judeo-Christian physicians. And he ends by repeating: "Plato should be your friend, and also Socrates; but truth should be a closer friend." Even the humorous variation he tells on the adage attests to its importance in Castro. The little story, which hinges on the pun *Plato:plato* (*plato*, as Castro explains, means a silver vessel in Portuguese), relates to the subject of truth versus deception discussed earlier: a patient promises his physician a silver bowl (*plato*) if he is healed of his fever by the following day. As the physician checks the patient's arm a day later, the agreement turns into a test of his veracity; for, noticing that the fever persists, he says (pointing to the silver bowl): "I like *plato* much, but I prefer truth" (p. 250).

While this work is not an apology for Jewish medicine, we can grasp its emphasis on breadth if we keep in mind that it was written by a Portuguese Jew who came to settle in Hamburg. We must consider the conditions under which Castro practiced medicine there. There is some question whether the senate realized from the beginning that Castro (or possibly any of the Portuguese immigrants in his group) were not Christian. By the time this work was written, however, no one had any doubts. We do not know whether the Lutheran preachers who railed against the Jewish settlements also specifically and immediately targeted the Jewish physician. Castro, who treated dukes and princes and whose services to the city were so much appreciated that he was the first and for many years the only Jew to be allowed to own a house in the center of Hamburg, speaks strongly on the subject of physicians as targets of calumny, as if from personal experience: "For there is hardly any human profession more exposed to this calamity" (p. 112). This may have a stronger emphasis than the point would have in most physicians (but not stronger than in De Pomis), although to separate the historical from the generically typical (from classical medicine onward) may be difficult.[45]

As a result of Castro's attempt to justify the profession of the physician to the Hamburg senate, his *Medicus-Politicus* has two potentially inconsistent characteristics. On the one hand the work may be called secular, laicistic, generally humanitarian—as when Castro insists that in a case of serious illness it is "useful and necessary" to give medication, while merely conceding that it is also "best" (*optimum*) to please God first. (Of course writers on medical ethics from Roman Catholic regions invariably discuss the question whether the physician is even allowed to undertake a cure without the patient first confessing to a priest or without urging the patient to confession, since the Church had laid down particular rules about that.) As we will be able to judge better in the next section, Castro advocates an unusually humanitarian treatment of enemies, presenting as a model of ethical behavior his maternal uncle Rodrigo Vaëz, a physician who treated the King of Fez although he was the enemy, embroiled in a war with Portugal. But on the other hand the book is also at least in part a state ethics; i.e. the perspective adopted is that of the ruling political body and assumes that body's right to diagnose the private body. As a result, the interest in *Medicus-Politicus* often merges with that of an incipient forensic medicine, as in the example of the Spanish sailors pretending to be ill, unwilling to board the ships of the Armada, or in the case narrated of a prostitute simulating a miscarriage in order to be found too weak to be sent out of town (pp. 251–52). To the modern reader, the most striking example of this kind is bk. 4, chap. 13, entitled *"Declarandi ratio circa emptitios servos"* (Method of Diagnosing Bought Servants), where Castro says: "All nations, except the northern ones, use bought servants, in whose purchase and sale they expect the counsel of the physician so that they know whether they are healthy or ailing" (p. 263).

But in case there should be any doubt about how this physician will decide if faced with a conflict he might perceive between duties of the state and medical duties, his discussion of the physician's obligation toward those traditionally and conventionally unworthy of care resolves it in an interesting way.

May the Physician Withhold His Service?

Of the large number of topics treated in the *Medicus-Politicus* I am for two reasons selecting for discussion an issue treated in bk. 3, chap. 15, "Whether the Physician may refuse help to someone requesting it": in this chapter Rodrigo a Castro, whose preface says the book is a novel and arduous endeavor, makes one of the few references to a Renaissance work of medical ethics; secondly, our previous discussion of De Pomis's stand on this controversial issue may supply some context for Castro's strong opinion on it (although Castro never mentions the Italian apologist for Jewish physicians).

The chapter begins by saying that as physicians almost all agree, not only those who have not called the physician and do not expect him are not to be visited, but the physician can legitimately neglect some who do seek his help: he can refuse his helping hand to some. Foremost among the latter, according to this view, are personal and general enemies (*inimici et hostes*) because he should avoid suspicion in case something happens "after the manner of men" (*humanitus*), but also certain friends, namely those known to be intemperate and never to listen to the doctor's prescriptions; next, one should not treat "barbarians" nor any people holding the art of medicine and its rules in contempt—a notion that bespeaks its classical heritage; finally the physician should not attempt to cure himself nor anyone close to him, since his objectivity would be in jeopardy.

Castro's claim that this is a near consensus of all physicians appears to be correct, as could be shown from incidental remarks in Renaissance commentaries on the Hippocratic oath. Instead, I merely point to Julius Alexandrinus (or Alessandri, 1506–1590), personal physician to Ferdinand I and Maximilian II as well as author of a book on the education and the duties of a physician, *De medicina et medico* (1557), who makes a point of warning against extending medical care to those unworthy of it.

For Alexandrinus, or rather his spokesman Turranus in an imagined dialogue, Hippocrates serves as the model physician for his thesis that medical help should not be given to bad people (*mali*), unworthy human beings (*perditi*), and to enemies.[46] Hippocrates' refusal to cure in one of these conditions becomes for him a sign of the ancient physician's generosity of mind (*generosus animus*), since he fearlessly spurned the request of a king and promise of rich reward, denying medical help to the most powerful of the barbarians and the enemy of all Greeks. Similarly, those who in modern times devote themselves to curing Turks, Alexandrinus argues, and (as some reports have it) are executed for lack of success, get their due deserts for their stupidity and greed. The physician has no legitimate duty toward Scyths, barbarians, toward any savage nation (*natio ulla effera*) that does not know the practice of medicine, nor to bandits (*latrones*) or other disgraced people. "Then the physician will deny help to someone seeking it?" asks Marcus, the other dialogue partner. "Indeed," replies Turranus and refers once more to the father of medicine. "For otherwise generosity (*liberalitas*) would forthwith lose its name so that it is generosity no more, when bestowed on the unworthy."[47] Medical care should not be provided without discrimination, for if it is given without distinction to the most abject people (*perditissimi homines*), the physicians will turn out to be the greatest evildoers. Marcus is overwhelmed by these arguments: "Then I have been wrong in this a long time, since I used to agree with Aristotle saying somewhere, if I remember correctly, that our purpose is only to cure, without any consideration of what may come of that beyond this end."[48] He adds that according to this old line of argument, we do not see someone constructing a house give much thought to whether the house will be put to good or bad uses, or the shoemaker much concerned with the purposes of the shoes or the caterer whether his culinary art will contribute to health or not. "But now I realize from you that medicine must look farther to purposes beyond its [immediate] end, purposes to which it accommodates its work or which it rejects."[49] I have given more than a minimal context of Alexandrinus's view in order to show that refusal of medical help to some people is an application of conceptions of medicine that in some ways may seem laudatory and truly farsighted. It would not be the first or last time in the history of medicine that ambitious ethical aims lead to obnoxious results.

Alexandrinus thought that for the idea of selectiveness of medical care he was on solid ground since he had Hippocrates, the father of medicine, on his side. The passage referred to is part of what in the Renaissance was taken to be Hippocrates' correspondence with various spokespersons for King Artaxerxis. (According to some modern historians, the entire volume of correspondence on a variety of subjects, including Hippocrates' famous account of visiting Democritus at Abdera, is a piece of imaginative literature, possibly the first epistolary novel.) The letters show the Persian king attempting to enlist Hippocrates' aid against the plague and being rebuffed by the physician. Hippocrates is said to have written to the governor of the Hellespont: "It is not proper that I should enjoy Persian opulence or save Persians from disease, since they are enemies of the Greeks. Be well."[50]

Thus, although, as Kibre points out,[51] the group of letters to which this one belongs was not available to the West until the fifteenth century, Castro is opposing what must have been to him a quite formidable tradition when he says: "Besides, I think, barbarian and intemperate people, however boorish, truculent, ill bred, and unused to remedies, should not at all be excluded from the benefits of medicine. To deny them medication would be similar to not teaching children the elements of writing because they irritate their teachers."[52] He goes on to point out that the notion of who is a "barbarian" is, like people's habits, subject to change, and that in his own time medicine is flowering among peoples (*gentes*) who took no notice of it during the time of Hippocrates and Galen. "Therefore I cannot see how such a wise and elegantly learned man as Julius Alexandrinus could hold that one should absolutely deny help to the enemy. For if we stretch out our hand to someone vanquished, though armed against us, when he asks for our mercy and we save his life, since with great minds humaneness toward the vanquished wins out and the praise of moderation and kindness is the more remarkable when reason for anger is most justified, it does not seem consonant with humaneness and reason that one should refuse help to someone asking for it."[53]

Castro calls Alexandrinus's argument—that the word "generosity" thus loses its proper meaning—"specious." Acknowledging that Alexandrinus is drawing on Hippocrates' resistance to the lure of lavish reward from Artaxerxis, he entirely agrees with Aristotle's argument that all arts and sciences have their immediate purpose to achieve and not any ulterior motive beyond that purpose; therefore the physician's aim is to bring about health. (In our later chapter on the ethics of curing contagious diseases, particularly syphilis, we will see the Italian Sitoni subject this position to a powerful critique.) Castro says: "Our medicine, which we have wanted to conjoin with probity and goodness, always aims at health as some good. For one should really ask what good purpose total destruction might serve for the leaders of our state: for while good ends do not justify ill means, cruelty is in itself an ill."[54] He adds that one should rather attempt to pacify enemies by doing them good, thus making them less hostile and ultimately turning them into friends.

The examples by which he then illustrates wise leaders of state acting in a humanitarian way include the following: Charles V ordering the captured son of the Duke of Saxony to be cured; his own uncle, Rodrigo Vaëz, with the knowledge of his king, John III of Portugal, treating the king of Fez, although he was an enemy; and the scriptures warning us not to spill the blood of war in peace. Castro insists that in his understanding anyone refusing to cure is a spiller of blood. He applies the precision of moral or legal casuistry to an imaginary case in which the leaders of state have forbidden a physician to give someone medical treatment: in that case, we are told, the physician sins not in curing, but in transgressing the edict (p. 167)—the assumption being, if I read the passage correctly, that Castro's ideal physician has no alternative.

Castro also makes some interesting distinctions regarding Hippocrates' refusal to fight the plague in Persia, the refusal that had been used by Alexandrinus and others to buttress their view of the physician's limited obligation. According to Castro, while Hippocrates was justified in refusing to neglect his friends and to pass over to the enemy for a price, if some individual Persians had implored him for help, he certainly would not have refused: for that would have been different from entirely abandoning his own and switching to the enemy. "Only one thing I ask: whoever it is requesting individual medical care, the physician should take that person up and attempt to cure that person with all diligence, whether Christian, Jew, Turk, or heathen; for all are linked by the law of *humanitas*, and *humanitas* requires that they all be treated equally by the physician."[55] This ringing statement of human equity and sameness of worth, as powerful as I have found anywhere in the medical literature of the period, is further supported by a denunciation (*impius error!*) of all those groups or peoples laying claim to some exclusivity and thereby raising themselves above others. While not specifically naming the Jews (he uses only the historical "Athenians" and "Romans"), he says that anyone reading "the divine historian Moses" would understand that all human beings are blood relatives, linked by the bond of same kind—another stimulus for a physician to treat all with the same diligence. "Indeed, to remove all suspicion, I do not know what more care and solicitude the adversary can be given so that we overcome whatever ill was in him by goodness."[56]

Although I have no evidence that Castro knew De Pomis's *Apologia*, there is no doubt in my mind that the Italian's book is the right context in which to see Castro's eloquent plea for humanitarian treatment of the enemy. We saw earlier that De Pomis, while denying that Jews and Christians were enemies, had to deal with the Christians' perception that Jews were praying for their destruction as enemies. His disquisition on the humanitarian treatment of enemies grew out of the hypothetical question: What if Jewish physicians consider Christians their enemies? Of course because there may have been some similarity between a Jewish physican's predicament in northern Italy and Castro's plight in Hamburg (as a Portuguese and as a Jew, very much the "other"), it is just as possible that Castro arrived at similar conclusions and equally strong convictions independently.

The tone of these two physicians treating similar subject matter is quite different: De Pomis's humanitarian ideas are admittedly and overtly linked to the plight of Jewish doctors; they are not disinterested, but in some sense limited and even self-serving. Also they are communicated as a defense from the position of the victim, a position of weakness. Castro's, by contrast, are meant to hold at the highest level of generality: his humanitarian view is that of a humanist freely speaking his mind and forcefully disagreeing with what he takes to be a powerful medical tradition, for which he makes Alexandrinus, an important author, the spokesman. While Castro's real situation as a Jewish physician may have been just as tenuous, the stance he adopts is that of a physician, not of a Jewish physician. Finally, Castro's pathos in some of the last sentences quoted, a pathos quite unusual in *Medicus-Politicus*, seems to be animated by firm conviction or, rather, experience: that grasping the hand of a human being asking for medical help in fact overcomes hostility.

The Physician's Defense:
Cure of the Body, Not of the Mind

Many of the Jewish doctors from Portugal were highly successful in their profession: Montalto, mentioned in my quotation from the contemporary *Mercure françois*, was granted by the French queen mother the unique privilege of practicing Judaism openly in France.[57] But although Montalto was so highly reputed that he was offered medical chairs at Bologna, Messina, and Pisa (where he would have succeeded the famous Mercuriale), there is evidence that he declined these positions for fear of religious persecution. As Friedenwald reports, "even after his death, his name figured largely in the *cause célèbre* which ended in the execution of the Queen's favorite" (p. 129). His notoriety as the religious "other" also speaks in the news clipping with which I opened this chapter.

Before Montalto, one of the most famous émigré physicians was Amatus Lusitanus, who in 1553 published a famous work on Dioscorides under the name of Johannes Rodericus Castelli Albi Lusitanus. It would seem that after dropping his baptized name, Amatus Lusitanus wore his Portuguese, and by implication Jewish, provenance like a badge or trademark. Born in 1511 of parents who seem to have been forced to convert to Christianity, he, like Montalto and a Castro a few years later, received his medical doctorate at Salamanca, practiced medicine in Portugal, but emigrated for fear of new waves of persecutions of baptized Jews. After staying six years in Antwerp, he became professor of medicine at Ferrara. While trying to obtain the position of city physician at Ragusa, he was accused of crypto-Judaism, lost his property by confiscation, and escaped imprisonment only by fleeing (1555) first to Pesaro, then (1556) to Ragusa, and eventually (1558) to Salonichi. He lived in Turkey, where he was able to profess Judaism openly, until his death (the date of which is unknown). The accolades this physician and distinguished anatomist received are extraordinary, and yet his professional career was obviously stinted by charges of Judaizing.

In an important essay entitled "Science in the Italian Universities in the Sixteenth and Early Seventeenth Centuries" (1975), Charles B. Schmitt traces the origin of the academic study of botany as it developed in conjunction with the study of medicine. But it would seem that on the basis of correspondence of Renaissance botanists he paints a somewhat too rosy, if not utopian, picture of the relationship among early botanists across religious and national divides:

> In all of these [letters] we see a dedicated determination to advance scientific knowledge and to exchange ideas and botanical specimens freely, with there being little evidence of envy, of competing interests or of national and religious differences.[58]

The relationship of two important botanist physicians, Pietro Andrea Mattioli (1500–1577) and Amatus Lusitanus, both writers of highly acclaimed commentaries on Dioscorides, is an important counter example, and it is in print, since Mattioli published his *Apologia adversus Amatum Lusitanum cum censura in eiusdem enarratione* in 1558. (It is also contained in his *Opera omnia*.) By its public nature the work may be an important index of how a competing botanist could be addressed by an Italian physician who, trained at Padua, had gained such fame through his learned work on Dioscorides that he became the personal physician of two emperors, Ferdinand and Maximilian II.

In his ill-tempered apology, written from Vienna (and dated 1557), Mattioli accuses Amatus, who claimed he had amended or corrected some errors made by Mattioli, of twenty "calumnies." Since my interest is not botany, I am not concerned with the specifics of Mattioli's allegations, but only the general tone of his piece, peppered with accusations of ingratitude, inhumanity, plagiarism, lack of learning, hallucinations, and arrogance. His conclusion is summarized in the margin, in the following outline-topic form: "[Amatus] Lusitanus is half Jewish (*Semi Iudaeus*). The Spaniards call such people Marranos, whom they despise extremely. About the reason why Amatus should struggle in blindness."[59] A small portion of the conclusion, which directly addresses Amatus, will suggest its flavor:

> Now it is enough for me to crush your calumnies. If I give satisfaction to them in your opinion also, I rejoice much for your sake. But if you persist in remaining as they say you are, certainly the judgment, the frank and fair opinion of everyone, will not depend on your unlearned and rash malevolence. Old gentility tells us that those who intruded into the sacrifices for the great goddess were immediately struck with blindness, where not so much blindness of sight as of insight is intended. But if I call you blind, Amatus, I am not impelled so much by pagan superstitious belief that you might meddle with the mysteries of some Cybele, but only for the reason that (as you experienced just recently) you turn away most perfidiously from the immortal God. For as I hear, first you make yourself of our religion, then you wholeheartedly adopt the Jewish laws and superstitions, and thus you offend not only human society but even the Most High; no wonder if you become untrue to yourself and lose any stability of mind. For not only is there no piety left in you, no religion, but even in the medical art, which you undeservedly profess, you are struck with blindness.[60]

This is public discourse in Roman Catholic territory in the sixteenth century, some forty years before the tightened hold of the Inquisition forced Montalto and a Castro to leave the Iberian Peninsula. (The exact date of Montalto's emigration is unknown.)

Rodrigo a Castro came to settle in Protestant Hamburg where, as I mentioned before, he was so successful a physician that he was allowed, by a special exemption in a contract (1617) between the Portuguese Jews and the Hamburg senate, to own a house in the Wallstrasse.[61] The king of Denmark, the Archbishop of Bremen, and the duke of Holstein were among his patients. His son Benedict (or Baruch Nehemias), who called himself *Lusitanus* in his publications although he was born in Hamburg in 1597, became the personal physician of Queen Christina of Sweden.

But to any reader of Luther's sharp piece *On the Jews and their Lies* (1543), which called for the burning of their synagogues, it will not come as a surprise that the position of Jews and, by implication, of Jewish physicians was also tenuous in Protestant countries (even though Hsia reminds us that the youthful Luther had written a compassionate pamphlet in 1523 with the title, "That Jesus Christ Was a Born Jew").[62] A thesis on political theory and recommended practice of the first decade of the seventeenth century (presided by Johann Gerhard at Jena), *Centuria quaestionum politicarum*, can serve as an index to the climate in a Lutheran academy. The first part of *decas 9*, section 1, devoted to the question "whether synagogues should be permitted in Christian states," acknowledges, in a manner that would have appeared urbane and balanced, that the Jews live peacefully among Christians and do not disparage Christianity despite some disquieting rumors, as, for instance, that of the yearly ritual slaying of a Christian child at Easter. Historians of the Jewish settlement in Hamburg have not noticed that this work may have been the reason why the Hamburg senate asked the University of Jena for advice (in 1611) when considering giving the Portuguese colony in Hamburg a permanent legal status.[63] For the general context, we also should remember that typically Protestants did not allow Catholic places of worship; in fact, the Emperor Ferdinand II complained to the Hamburg senate (in 1627) that in the Hanseatic city Jews had more religious freedom than his coreligionists.[64]

Even more important in my context than the candidate's view on freedom of worship (he ultimately denied it to the Jews) is his discussion of Jewish physicians: in section 5, devoted to state regulation of medicine, the candidate, Paul Trane from Stavanger, Norway, proposes that, together with *uromantes* and magicians, "Jewish physicians are rightly to be disallowed, considering that no physician in Germany, Bohemia or Hungary has yet met a Mesue, Avicenna, Galen, or Hippocrates; but only after they have been destroyed by debauchery, they devote themselves to medicine and, according to Ant. Ma[r]gar., writing in German about the beliefs of the Jews, they are thought to kill *Goïm* licitly."[65] The reference is to the book *Der gantz jüdish Glaub* ([Augsburg], 1530) by Antonius Margarita, who on the last pages of the book calls himself a recent convert to Christianity. This account of Jewish ceremonies and habits (illustrated by numerous woodcuts) by someone presenting himself as a former insider was a mainstay of Renaissance anti-Jewish propaganda. No doubt Luther was familiar with it; von Hörnigk, whom I will discuss next, refers to it several times.

In the first decades of the century (when Rodrigo a Castro was writing his *Medicus-Politicus*, and continuing into the thirties), there seems to have been a groundswell of detraction, economically or religiously motivated, against Jewish doctors in Germany. Some of the publications in this vein were anonymous and of limited distribution, and are therefore difficult to find today. There is, for instance, the book by a Frankfurt physician, Ludwig von Hörnigk (1600–1667), *Medicaster Apella oder Juden Artzt* (Strassburg, 1631), a general attack on Jewish physicians. (*Apella*, as Du Cange's *Glossarium infimae Latinitatis* explains, means *quasi sine pelle*, "as if without skin," i.e. "circumcised Jew," and seems always to have been a disparaging term.) Von Hörnigk is the same author who also wrote, as I mentioned before, a book entitled *Politia medica* (1638), the title of which, as I suspected earlier, may stand in some filiation with Castro's *Medicus-Politicus* and may even have contributed to paving the way for the later acceptance of the term *ärztliche Politik* (in the specific medical sense of medical *oeconomia*). If that is so, Hörnigk's relationship to Rodrigo a Castro presents an interesting problem. Friedenwald says only of Rodrigo's son Benedict: "Neither [Benedict] De Castro nor Hörnigk mentions the other's name."[66] While this is factually correct, it is not the entire story.

At the beginning of his book *Medicaster Apella*, before he launches into his diatribe against Jews, von Hörnigk imagines the art of medicine as a beautiful tree with many branches: the branches are the developments of medicine in different countries represented by the names of outstanding physicians in them, Italians, Germans, etc. Among physicians from the Iberian peninsula, i.e. "unter den Portugalesern und Spaniern," he lists (I am preserving his spelling) Fonseca, Amatus Lusitanus, Nunnius, Rod. de Castro, Steph. Rod. Castrensis, Thomas a Veiga Valverda—apparently without realizing that they are New Christians, Marranos, or Jews, or certainly without making an issue of it. The main prong of von Hörnigk's attack is against one Doctor Schlamm of Frankfurt, who is presented as ignorant. Because the front rows of university anatomical theaters like that in Padua are reserved for Christian students, von Hörnigk tells us, Jews have never seen "where the *calor nativus* and *balsamum naturale* reside and what the *humores* are really like" (p. 148). Jews are presented as hating Christians and praying for their destruction, and as poisoning their rulers (pp. 74, 201, and 213). From Schlamm and a few other local Frankfurt physicians (one Simon Wageman and a

Jacob Benaker from Constantinople), who are presented as impostors, he generalizes to all Jewish physicians. The distinguishing feature of the *Judenarzt* is said to be duplicity: his friendly talk and smiling face hide an evil heart, a particularly destructive version of dissimulation. Please understand, von Hörnigk says, addressing the reader, "that the Jew has no affection or love for you, that he feels only jealous and hostile toward you."[67]

Did von Hörnigk not realize that Rodrigo a Castro was Jewish, or did he exempt the famous Lusitani physicians from his attack? Some such explanation might hold for this work by von Hörnigk, and could be confirmed by a reading of much of his later *Politia medica* (1638), written when the author had become *physicus ordinarius* in the city of Frankfurt. The long subtitle, which I cite in the notes, indicates that *politia* refers at least in part to the policing of medicine.[68] But in the opening pages (on the comportment of the physician), von Hörnigk many times refers to Rodrigo a Castro's *Medicus-Politicus*, and always for support and in agreement—on page 6 alone there are three such references. In the same work, von Hörnigk will not only refer to his *Medicaster Apella* but launch into a similar disquisition against Jewish physicians (barred from practice, as he admiringly reports, by the city laws of Mainz).[69] Is it possible that even at this date, i.e. after publication of an apology for Jewish doctors by Rodrigo's son Benedict (which we will consider below), the author was either ignoring or exempting the "Portuguese"? This seemed to me the only possible explanation until I came upon a sentence in *Politia medica* that points to the deviousness and craft of this author. Unfortunately I cannot find the keyword in it, *Protugaleser*, in any dictionary. From the context, however, it would be a variant of the *Portugaleser* ("Portuguese") quoted earlier and in this sentence would mean, "Portuguese gold coin": "Henceforth [Jewish physicians] should not be allowed or permitted [to practice] any more, no matter how impressively their patrons speak for them, of whom some perhaps allow themselves to be bribed with *protugaleser*, rings, and other deceiving gifts or else are in league with them in commerce or barter."[70] In the German context, the charge of venality of patrons could only refer to the contract with the Hamburg senate and the Portuguese Jewish community (consisting primarily of merchants), among whom the Castros were the most prominent physicians. Since Rodrigo a Castro had died in 1627, this indirect calumny was aimed at his sons (two of whom were physicians). By that time von Hörnigk could have had the dubious reputation of being the foremost attacker of Jewish physicians, and thus may have received information about Hamburg from a local physician there. In fact, such information was in print.

The Hamburg physician Jacob Martini (not to be confused with his famous namesake, a professor at Wittenberg), in a work whose title is so close to von Hörnigk's as to suggest filiation, *Apella medicaster bullatus oder Judenarzt*, presents the image of a Jewish doctor who goes to great lengths of malicious pretense to gain access to Christians. (Here again is the topic of dissimulation as an anti-Jewish charge.) In the subtitle the purpose of the book is programmatically given as contrasting a Jewish physician "per antithesin" to a Christian doctor. Martini's main example is Rodrigo a Castro, who he claims first pretended a desire to become part of the Christian community and had some of his children baptized, but later openly professed Judaism.[71]

While Martini's book is unquestionably motivated by professional envy (in his prefatory letter to the reader the author acknowledges that "many a patient in his illness sends rather for a Portuguese Jewish physician than a Christian" [sig. Aiv]), it is broadly based on the kind of Protestant thought that Hsia describes, indicated by references to Luther's book on Jews (p. 4), Buxdorf's *Judenschul*, and even Melanchthon's argument that in the physical sciences dubious points can be resolved by referring to divine authority—a most questionable application of Melanchthon's views on natural law (see my chapter 1). But Martini also knows Ludwig von Hörnigk, and David de Pomis's defense of Jewish physicians as well as that of Benedict a Castro. Unlike von Hörnigk, this Hamburg physician openly aims his barbs at Portuguese doctors, asking with malicious irony how it could happen that such presumably saintly Portuguese physicians were evicted by the Lusitani (pp. 74–75). As to the charge made by Von Hörnigk that Jews overcharge their patients, Martini reluctantly admits that "our lousy Jews, i.e. our Portuguese (*Lusitanos dico*)," may act a little more professionally (p. 124). His central argument is to expose as "calumny" the view that requiring a physician to have *pietas* represents a confusion of theology and medicine (p. 130). To claim that the physician's business is medicine, not conscience, would mean that he is without conscience, *gewissenlos* (p. 166). Martini would like to "invert" such a claim: a physician is concerned not only with what relates to medicine and health, but what relates *ad bonam conscientiam*—and as a person of ill repute, the Jewish doctor cannot have such (p. 165). As Martini indicates by his use of the word "calumny" and by the direction of his central argument, he is here quarreling with Benedict a Castro's eloquent Latin defense of Jewish physicians *Flagellum calumniantium* (Amsterdam, 1631).

Published under the pseudonym Philotheus Castellus, this work by Rodrigo's son, now very rare, is important in my context because it spins out a powerful argument for what I would like to call secular medicine. Its full title indicates that it is in fact conceived as an apologia specifically for "Lusitani" physicians.[72] The apology, according to Hans Schröder, may have been occasioned by an attack by the Hamburg physician Joachim Curtius (1585–1642), whose *Exhortatio* I have so far been unable to locate.[73] Since Benedict a Castro refers to the calumniator as an *anonymus*, Curtius's work would have had to circulate in some other form (anonymously and probably in German) before 1631. Castro refers to the title of a denigrating work as *Freudiger Wecker* (p. 95), which may be the first version of the *Exhortatio*.

As part of the paratextual material, so often bulging in works of the period, Benedict a Castro's *Flagellum calumniantium* contains a long letter by Abraham Zacuto complimenting the younger physician on undertaking the task of defending Jewish physicians. Then follows a letter to Benedict by someone calling himself Philaletes Lusitanus, pointing out that there is a tradition of Christian emperors holding Jewish physicians in high esteem. The author of that letter, identifying himself as having received his doctorate *in Complutensi Academia* (Alcalá de Henares, near Madrid) but otherwise unknown, then responds to the charge that Jewish physicians corrupt their Christian patients' souls: "What? Physicians do not concern themselves with conscience, with the health of the soul, but the health of the body and the remedy and cure of diseases, and thus he [the anonymous writer] should have found fault with Jewish physicians not for their Jewishness (for that is a question of religion), but for some supposed lack of learning and an ineptitude for the art of medicine."[74]

Benedict a Castro picks up individual arguments of the person he calls the "anonymous" attacker (Curtius?)—as, for instance, what seems to have been a commonplace of anti-Jewish propaganda through the ages, that Jews (and therefore Jewish physicians) curse the Christian religion. Of course he calls the allegation false (p. 5), which will not keep von Hörnigk from repeating it with new anecdotes (p. 201). But his key argument understandably is a version of the one quoted above from the Portuguese Philaletes' prefatory letter, namely that there is no necessary connection between medicine and Christianity. Here Benedict a Castro does not mince words: "For example, if I should ask you why you practice the art of medicine, you would say without doubt, because as a doctor you are a Christian. But this assertion is stupid and of no moment," and he adduces "divine Hippocrates" (as a non-Christian) to support his point.[75] Benedict a Castro also recognizes that the seemingly devout Jew-baiters are not the best physicians in Germany: "Why have the most famous German physicians (among whom the most learned Sennert takes first place) never supported such an argument, which slanders good people?"[76]

For the history of medical ethics, the contribution of some Lusitani physicians was to make a powerful argument for secular medicine or, as the French might put it, *une médicine laïque.* The programmatic goal of medicine became, sometimes as a reaction to anti-Jewish attack, to treat the body rather than the soul. While implicitly and sometimes explicitly this was a medicine perceived as useful to the state, we also saw that Rodrigo a Castro, on a matter for several reasons highly important to him, namely the medical treatment of enemies, differentiates between his medical and his civic duties and leaves little doubt about how he would resolve a dilemma. In the writings of exiled Portuguese physicians, we can see the formation of what in the eighteenth century will be medical and ethical commonplaces. While we may now feel uneasy with some of the ideas—such as separating body from spirit (or psyche), or the civic from the medical—and may recognize them as inordinately pat, historians will have to give these physicians in their extraordinary predicament the credit for creating something that can be called *medical* ethics, rather than a general (and usually Christian) ethics applied to medical practice.

NOTES

1. *La Continuation du Mercure françois ou Suitte de l'Histoire de l'Auguste Régence de la Royne Marie de Medicis, sous son fils . . . Louis XIII* (Paris, 1613), p. 5.

2. *Mercure françois. Quatriesme tôme, ou Les mémoires de la suitte de l'Histoire de notre temps* (Paris, 1617), pp. 45–46. On Montalto, see Harry Friedenwald, "Montalto: A Jewish Physician at the Court of Marie de Medicis and Louis XIII," *Bulletin of the Institute of Historical Medicine,* 3 (1935): 129–58.

3. Ludovicus Lemos, in the biography he wrote for Zacuto's *Opera omnia* (1642), as quoted in Harry Friedenwald, *Jews and Medicine: Essays*, 2 vols. (Baltimore: Johns Hopkins Press, 1944), vol. 1, (pp. 307–321), p. 310.

4. Hans Schröder, *Lexikon der hamburgischen Schriftsteller* (Hamburg, 1851), entry 581 (De Castro, Roderich); see also Joachim Whaley, *Religious Toleration and Social Change in Hamburg, 1529–1819* (Cambridge: Cambridge University Press, 1985). On the relationship between Sephardim in Holland and in Hamburg, see Jonathan I. Israel, *Empires and Entrepots: The Dutch, The Spanish Monarchy, and the Jews, 1585–1713* (London and Roncevert, W.V.: Hambledon, 1990).

5. *Medicus-Politicus* (1614 ed.), p. 25 (simulation of illness); p. 276 (music); *De universa mulierum medicina* (Hamburg, 1603), pars 2, lib. 4, chap. 17, p. 314 (for post-partum depression or, rather, post-partum melancholy).

6. Friedenwald, *Jews in Medicine* vol. 2, pp. 448–49 : "The Doctors de Castro," particularly p. 451n. Joachim Whaley has only one sentence on our physician: *Religious Toleration and Social Change in Hamburg*, p. 75. One of the earliest suggestions that Castro first pretended he wanted to be part of the Christian community and that he had some of his children baptized (which is far from certain) is in the anti-Jewish diatribe by the Hamburg physician Jacob Martini, *Apella medicaster bullatus oder Judenarzt* (Hamburg, 1636), p. 100.

7. Yoseph Hayim Yerushalmi, *From Spanish Court to Italian Ghetto: Isaac Cardoso; A Study in Seventeenth-Century Marranism and Jewish Apologetics* (New York and London: Columbia University Press, 1971) and Perez Zagorin, *Ways of Lying: Dissimulation, Persecution and Conformity in Early Modern Europe* (Cambridge, Mass.: Harvard University Press, 1990).

8. Quoted from Yerushalmi, *From Spanish Court to Italian Ghetto*, p. 64; also Zagorin, *Ways of Lying*, p. 56.

9. David B. Ruderman, *A Valley of Vision: The Heavenly Journey of Abraham Yagel* (Philadelphia: University of Pennsylvania Press, 1990), p. 3, and *Kabbalah, Magic, and Science: The Cultural Universe of a Sixteenth-Century Jewish Physician* (Cambridge, Mass: Harvard University Press, 1988). On the relationship between popes and Jews, and particularly Paul IV's bull "Cum nimis absurdum" (1555), see also the entry "popes" in the *Encyclopedia Judaica* (Jerusalem: Keter, 1972–82), cols. 851–61.

10. *Medicus-Politicus*, p. 2 : ". . . proposi tum hoc egregium, quod vix quisquam ante hac tentare ausus fuit." Later, perhaps by what may be called a *topos modestiae* (and, interestingly, in a letter prefaced to a work by Zacutus), he was to call the book "a toy of his old age" (*fuit lusus senectutis; Zacuto, De Medicorum principum historia* [Lyon, 1642], sig. c5ᵛ).

11. Antonio Hernández Morejón, *Historia bibliográfica de la medicina española*, 7 vols. (Madrid, 1842–52), vol. 3, p. 387: "Nunca será esta preciosa obra bastantamente encomiada. . . ." Lope de Vega's sonnets are printed in Henriques' *Retrato del perfecto médico* (Madrid, 1595).

12. *Medicus-Politicus*, p. 89.

13. Hernández Morejón, *Historia bibliográfica*, vol. 3, p. 165. The sonnet is quoted there.

14. Henriques, *Retrato del perfecto médico* p. 184.

15. Zagorin, (*Ways of Lying*, pp. 32–33), summarizing "Ad IIII Regum Cap. V," in *Textus Bibliae cum glossa ordinaria, Nicolai de Lyra Postilla* . . . (Basel, 1508).

16. In addition to the place quoted, Zagorin refers to Naaman on pp. 69, 73, 102, 104, 109, 110–11, 136, 138, 139, 140, 144–45, 146, 147, 151, 223, 237, 244, 284, 327.

17. *Republic*, bk. 3, 329B; Loeb ed., vol. 1, p. 213. Plato says that "we must surely prize truth most highly. For if we were right in what we were just saying, and falsehood is in very deed useless to the gods, but to men useful as a remedy or form of medicine, it is obvious that such a thing must be assigned to the physicians, and laymen should have nothing to do with it. . . ." For Jacques Derrida's far-reaching discussion of Plato's use of the word *pharmakon* in other works, see *La dissémination* (Paris: Seuil, 1972).

18. In the nineteenth century, the German term for this range of concerns was still "ärztliche Politik." As we shall see later, however, von Hörnigk also intends by his title the policing of medicine.

19. R. Bandeira, "La renaissance et l'Ecole Iatroéthique Portugaise du XVIe siècle," in *Atti, XXI Congresso internationale di Storia della Medicina (1988)*, ed. Raffaele A. Bernabeo (Bologna: Monduzzi, 1988) pp. 675–81: ". . . tout un ensemble de nouveaux donnés conçus par les Découvertes et diffusés par l'Humanisme portugais dans l'Europe et, à partir de la fin du XVIe siècle consolidés dans la conjoncture hispanique de l'époque" (p. 680).

20. Ibid. "Parallèlement, il y a eu une émigration médicale importante de médecins portugais vers divers pays de l'Europe, non avec des buts universitaires ou d'enseignement, mais assistencielles (*sic*), ceux-la mêmes impregnés des idées de l'époque et profondement intégrés des idées medicales Renaissantes."

21. Stephen Gilman, *The Spain of Fernando de Rojas: The Intellectual Landscape of La Celestina* (Princeton, N.J.: Princeton University Press, 1972), p. 27.

22. The works are summarized and excerpted by Harry Friedenwald, "The Apologetic Works of Jewish Physicians," in his *Jews and Medicine* vol. 1, pp. 31–38. On Isaac Cardoso (*ca.* 1604–1680) who is a little late for my focus, see Yerushalmi, *From Spanish Court to Italian Ghetto*.

23. *The Examination of Mens Wits*, trans. R[ichard] C[arew] (London, 1594), pp. 183–85.

24. M. K. Reed, *Juan Huarte de San Juan* (Boston: Twayne, 1981), p. 23.

25. See Américo Castro, *The Spaniards: An Introduction to Their History*, trans. W. F. King and S. Margaretten (Berkeley: University of California Press, 1971), p. 547 and *The Structure of Spanish History*, trans. E. L. King (Princeton, N.J.: Princeton University Press, 1954), p. 491: "It is well known that medicine was one of the professions most widely practiced by educated Jews, and most neglected by Spanish Christians. We rarely find physicians in the royal household who are not Jews, and when we do, they are Frenchmen." Cecil Roth writes about (Renaissance) Portugal: "Nearly all of the most illustrious physicians of the day were of Jewish origin, and many of them devout Jews at heart; the profession was indeed adopted by some persons specifically by

reason of the facilities which it afforded for the observance of the Sabbath." *A History of the Marranos* (Philadelphia: The Jewish Publication Society of America, 1947), p. 71. Also Yosef Hayim Yerushalmi, *From Spanish Court to Italian Ghetto*, p. 71: "The popularity of the medical profession among New Christians in Spain and Portugal was due to a variety of factors, among which the long and venerable tradition of Jewish medicine which lay behind them should not be ignored." I owe these references (and much of what I know about Iberian culture) to my generous colleague Samuel Armistead.

26. For the general context, see my *Melancholy, Genius, and Utopia in the Renaissance* (Wiesbaden: Harrassowitz, 1991).

27. Henriques, *Retrato del perfecto médico*, p. 146: ". . . porque para cosa tan alta no bastava ingenio natural, por subido que fuesse."

28. Ibid., p. 145.

29. Saint Antoninus, *Summa theologica*, pars 3 (Lyon, 1542), tit. 7, c. 2, paragraph 5: "Medici non admittuntur ad practicam artis nisi iurati et de legitimo matrimonio nati."

30. Reed, *Juan Huarte de San Juan*, p. 24. On a Jewish physician (in Italy) close to the tradition of the occultists, see David B. Ruderman, *Kabbalah, Magic, and Science*. In fact Rudermann sees Yagel as a Jewish *magus* of that generation (see p. 115).

31. David de Pomis, *De Medico hebraeo enarratio apologetica* (Venice, 1588), p. 72: "Vide (obsecro) de his, et aliis Iudaeis medicis, quid vulgari idiomate scripserit, Nicolaus Nicolai, Dominus artefevillae, Camerarius, et Geografus ordinarius Regis Galliae. Haec sit, in Thracia (vulgo Turchia) Constantinopoli praesertim, quamplures reperiuntur Turcae, qui medicam artem profitentur; illamque exercent. Sed multo plures Iudaei quam Turcae." For an account by a modern historian of the role of Sephardic Jews as physicians in the Middle East, see Bernard Lewis, *The Jews of Islam* (Princeton, N.J.: Princeton University Press, 1984), particularly pp. 130–31.

32. Friedenwald, "Apologetic Works of Jewish Physicians," in *Jews in Medicine;* vol. 1, pp. 31–53; p. 53 on calumniators.

33. *Enarratio apologetica*, p. 10: ". . . miseratione, quae naturaliter (ut modo dicebamus) hominibus inest."

34. Ibid.: "Si vero depressos curemus, humanitate utemur; nobis ipsis suadentes, omnes aequaliter in humanitatis serie esse insertos."

35. For a history of the Blood Libel, rejections of it by the Church, as well as accounts of horrifying punishments, see Yerushalmi, *From Spanish Court to Italian Ghetto*, pp. 455–68, and R. Po-Chia Hsia, *The Myth of Ritual Murder: Jews and Magic in Reformation Germany* (New Haven and London: Yale University Press, 1988).

36. *Enarratio apologetica*, p. 58: ". . . quia Iudaeus, et Christianus, parum inter se differre viduntur . . . Unum Deum colunt, eadem mirabilia simul confirmant. Eadem praecepta (traditionibus, ceremonialibusque exceptis) ut saepe iam dictum a nobis est, observant."

37. Ibid., p. 59: "Quare vel caeco perspicuum existere potest, quod Religionis diversitas, haud tam magna inter hebraeum, Christianumque sit qua scelus aliquod, in se ipsos, committere queant."

38. Ibid., p. 11: "Unum tamen, obiter dicere fas est numquam veram amicitiam temporis intervallo, aetate, Religionis discrimine, impediri aliquo modo posse."

39. R. Po-Chia Hsia, *The Myth of Ritual Murder*, p. 132.

40. *Enarratio apologetica*, p. 39: "Gentes externae, hoc est Gallicam, Germaniam, Hispaniam, Italiam, Europamque totam incolentes, vere inimici nostri non sunt, nec umquam fuerunt."

41. Ibid., p. 10: "inimici, aut physico amore affecti. Denuo aut eadem, aut diversa Religione praediti."

42. P. 10–11: "Si vero inimici sunt a nobis curandi, quod non minori cura eis opitulemur, pro comperto habendum; nihilque ambiguitatis est: nam, cum eorum vitam sponte nobis tradiderint, haud amplius inimici sunt nostri, quin potius amici prorsus evadunt: quos aliquo pacto laedere, nefas est, ac tanquam captivi, aut victi nobis habentur."

43. Herman Kellenbenz, *Sephardim an der unteren Elbe: Ihre wirtschaftliche Bedeutung vom Ende des 16. bis zum Ende des 18. Jahrhunderts* (Wiesbaden: Franz Steiner, 1958), p. 327.

44. *Medicus-Politicus*, p. 86: ". . . non enim religionem docet, sed medicinam. Amicus Plato, Amicus Socrates, magis amica veritas."

45. I cannot tell whether M. Kayserling has more than internal evidence when, in his biographical essay on Rodrigo a Castro, he says that response to calumny motivated him to write *Medicus-Politicus* ("Zur Geschichte der jüdischen Ärzte (II): Rodrigo a Castro," *Monatsschrift für Geschichte und Wissenschaft des Judenthums* 8 [1859]: 330–39; particularly p. 337).

46. Alessandrinus, *De medicina et medico* (Zürich, 1557), p. 130.

47. Ibid., p. 131: "Ergo cuidam medicum auxilium poscenti deerit medicus, ait tum Marcus? Deerit, inquit Turranus. . . . Et enim si liberalitas ipsa nomen statim suum amittit, ut liberalitas ulterius non sit, quae indignis confertur."

48. Ibid.: "Tum Marcus, longe, inquit, opinione mea falsus sum hactenus, qui crediderim artes, scientiasque, idque ex Aristotelis alicubi, si recte memini, sententia, finem semper suum solummodo curare, non admodum sollicitas si quid extra finem eveniat."

49. Ibid., p. 132: "Nunc autem longius, atque ultra finis sui terminos prospicere debere medicinam animadverto ex te, ut aliis operam suam accomodet, aliis neget."

50. Wesley D. Smith's translation in Hippocrates, *Pseudepigraphic Writings*, ed. W. D. Smith (Leiden and New York: Brill, 1990), p. 53. In the Littré ed., this is vol. 9, p. 317. On the Hippocratic pseudepigraphica, as Smith has called them (i.e. writings with false superscriptions), see Smith, *The Hippocratic Tradition* (Ithaca, N.Y., and London: Cornell University Press, 1979), p. 216, and Owsei Temkin, *Hippocrates in a World of Pagans and Christians* (Baltimore and London: Johns Hopkins University Press, 1991), pp. 57–75. Temkin's discussion of the legend of Hippocrates as a patriot is particular relevant to my argument.

51. See Pearl Kibre, *Hippocrates Latinus: Repertorium of Hippocratic Writings in the Latin Middle Ages*, rev. ed. (New York: Fordham University Press, 1985), p. 158.

52. *Medicus-Politicus*, p. 166: "Caeterum barbaros et intemperantes homines quantumvis agrestes, truculentos, incultosque, et remediis parum assuetos a beneficio medicinae nequaquam excludendos esse censemus: iis enim medicamenta denegare non aliud esset, quam pueros non instituere primis literarum elementis, quia interdum praeceptoribus irascantur."

53. Ibid.: "Neque etiam video, quomodo vir sapiens et eleganter eruditus, Julius Alexandrinus, hosti auxilium penitus denegandum esse adstruat: si enim ei, quem contra nos armatum vivimus victo tamen, ubi gratiam implorat, manum porrigimus, et vitam ipsius servamus, quia magnis animis adversus prostratos succedit humanitas, et tunc praecipua laus clementiae est et beneficentiae, cum irae causae sunt iustissimae: sane nec humanitati, nec rationi consonum videtur, ut auxilium implorantem destituas."

54. Ibid, p. 167: "Praesertim vero nostra haec medicina, quam probitatem et bonitatem conjunctam habere diximus, repicit semper sanitatem, ut bonum quiddam. An vero bono cessura sit ad eos, qui reipublicae praesunt, pertinet inquirere: neque vero facienda sunt mala, ut eveniant bona; est autem crudelitas per se malum."

55. Ibid., p. 168: "Sed id monemus, ut quemlibet particularem auxilium postulantem curandum suscipiat medicus, susceptumque omni sedulitate tractare studeat, sive Christianus ille sit, sive Judaeus, sive Turca, sive Gentilis: omnes enim humanitatis lege sunt colligati, et omnes pariter a medico tractandos esse humanitas postulat."

56. Ibid.: "Immo ut omnis suspicio removeatur, nescio quid plus curae ac sollicitudinis in adversario adhibendum, ut malitiam, si qua in eo fuerat, bonitate superemus."

57. Jonathan I. Israel, *Empires and Entrepots* p. 335; also Friedenwald, "Montalto," *Bull. Inst. Hist. Med.*, pp. 129–58.

58. Charles B. Schmitt, "Science in the Italian Universities in the Sixteenth and Early Seventeenth Centuries," in his *The Aristotelian Tradition and Renaissance Universities* (London: Variorum Reprints, 1984): essay xiv, p. 42.

59. Pietro Andrea Mattioli, *Apologia adversus Amathum cum censura*, in *Opera Omnia* (Frankfurt, 1608) p. 20: "Lusitanus Semi Iudaeus. Hispani tales maranos vocant quos maxime detestantur. Cur Amathus tanta laboret caecitate."

60. Ibid., "Nunc satis mihi est, si tuas contuderim calumnias, quibus si tuo quoque iudicio a me est satisfactum, vehementer tua causa gaudeo, sin is maneas, ac perseveres, qualem te esse praedicant, certe non omnium iudicum, candor, ac aequabilitas ex una tua indocta et praecipiti pendebit malevolentia. Narrat vetusta gentilitas eos, qui se intulissent magnae Deae sacrificiis, confestim excaecari, quam quidem caecitatem illi non tam ad oculos, quam ad mentem referebant. At ego Amathe non te ideo caecum dico ductus hac gentilium superstitione quod Cybeles alicuius te insereris sacris, sed ea tantum ratione, ac sententia (sit tu ipse iam pridem in te experiris) quod a Deo immortali perfidissime disciscas. Et enim (ut audio) nunc nostrae religionis

teipsum facias, nunc Iudaicis legibus superstitionibusque te totum addicas, et ita non solum in homines, sed in ipsum Deum Optimum Maximum insolescas, minime est mirum, si a te ipso quoque deficias, et omni statu mentis dimovearis. Ut non modo in te nulla vigeat pietas, nulla religio, verum et in ipsa medica facultate, quam immerito profiteris plurimum caecutias."

61. M. Isler quotes the relevant passage, see "Zur ältesten Geschichte der Juden in Hamburg," *Zeitschrift für hamburgische Geschichte* 6 (1875): 461–79; particularly p. 472.

62. R. Po-Chia Hsia, *The Myth of Ritual Murder* p. 133; but, as Hsia points out, Luther also believed that Jews practiced medicine in order to kill Christians (p. 132).

63. Alfred Feilchenfeld, "Anfang und Blüthezeit der Portugiesengemeinde in Hamburg," *Zeitschrift für hamburgische Geschichte* 10 (1899): 199–240; p. 205.

64. Ibid., pp. 216–17.

65. Johann Gerhard (praeses), *Centuria quaestionum politicarum*, respondente Paulo Trane Stavangrio Nortvego (2d ed., Jena, 1608), sig. N3v: "Improbandi merito Medici Judaei, praeterquam enim quod nullus Medicus in Germania, Bohemia, Ungaria vidit Mesuen, Avicenna, Galenum, Hippocratem, sed postquam omnia luxu obsumsere, Medicae arti fere se tradant, teste Ant. Ma[r]gar. in scripto Germ. de fide Jud. etiam licite se occidere Goïm arbitrantur."

66. Friedenwald, *Jews in Medicine*, vol. 1, p. 54n.

67. Ludwig von Hörnigk, *Medicaster Apella oder Juden Artzt* (Strassburg, 1631), p. 333: ". . . daß der Jud kein *affection* zu dir trägt, daß er dir mißgönstig und feind ist."

68. *Politia medica* oder Beschreibung dessen was die Medici, sowohl ins gemein als auch verordnete Hof- Statt- Feld- Hospital- und Pest-Medici, Apothecker, Materialisten, Wundtärtzt, Barbierer, Feldscherer, Oculisten, Bruch-und Steinschneider, Zuckerbecker, Krämer und Bader, desgleichen die obriste geschwohrne Frauwen, Hebammen, unter Frawen und Kranckenpflegere, Wie nicht weniger allerhandt unbefugte, betriegliche und angemaßte Aertzte, darunter alte Weiber, Beutelschneider, Crystallenseher, Dorffgeistliche, Einsiedler, Fallimentirer, Gauckler, Harnpropheten, Juden, Kälberärtzt, Landstreicher, Marctschreyer, Nachrichter, Ofenschwärmer, Pseudo-Paracelsisten, Quacksalber, Rattenfänger, Segensprecher, Teuffelsbander, Unholden, Waltheintzen, Ziegeuner, etc. / So dann endlichen / Die Patienten oder Krancke selbsten zu thun, und was, auch wie sie in Obdacht zu nehmen, Allen Herrn-Höfen, Republiken, und Gemeinden zu sonderbahrem Nutzen und guten / Aus H. Schrifft, Geist- und Weltlichen Rechten, Policey-Ordnungen und vielen bewehrten Schrifften zusammengetragen (Frankfurt, 1638).

69. *Politia medica*, pp. 178–83; on Mainz, p. 178. On other cities, see Moses A. Spira, "Meilensteine der jüdischen Ärzte in Deutschland," in *Melemata: Festschrift für Werner Leibbrand*, ed. Joseph Schumacher, Martin Schrenk, Jörn H. Wolf (Mannheim: Mannheimer Grossdruckerei, 1967): pp. 48–58.

70. Ibid., p. 183: ". . . und sollen billich nicht mehr gelitten oder geduldet werden, wie stattlich auch ihre Patronen die Worth thun, deren mancher vielleicht sich mit Protugalesern, Ringen, und andern bethörlichen Geschenken verblenden last, oder sonsten mit ihnen in Handlung und Schacherey steckt."

71. *Apella medicaster bullatus*, p. 100. Excerpts from this rare book (available at the library of the Ärztliche Verein, Hamburg) are printed by M. Isler, "Zur ältesten Geschichte der Juden in Hamburg," pp. 476–78. Isler gives the title of the work as *Apollo Medicaster bullatus*, which is a mistake. For the correct title of the work and its aim also to criticize Rodrigo a Castro's son Benedict, see also Hans Schröder, *Lexikon der hamburgischen Schriftsteller* (Hamburg, 1851), vol. 1, p. 516.

72. The full title is *Flagellum calumniantium seu apologia In qua Anonymi Cujusdam calumniae refutantur eiusdem mentiendi libido detegitur, Clarissimorum Medicorum legitima methodus commendatur, empericorum inscitia ac temeritas tamquam perniciosa Reipublicae damnatur.* Friedenwald (who translated an excerpt from a copy at Hamburg) knew of no copy in the United States (*Jews in Medicine*, vol. 1, p. 58). The Universitätsbibliothek Kiel and the British Library have copies. According to Friedrich Niewoehner, this is a translation of an earlier treatise *Tratado da Calumnia* (Antverp, 1629). See Niewoehner, *Veritas sive varietas: Lessings Toleranzparabel und das Buch Von den drei Betrügern* (Heidelberg: Lambert Schneider, 1988), p. 355. Also my essay, "The Contribution of Exiled Portuguese Jews in Renaissance Medical Ethics," in *Expulsion of the Jews: 1492 and After*, ed. Raymond B. Waddington and Arthur H. Williamson (New York and London: Garland, 1994), pp. 147–59.

73. Nor had Friedenwald found it. For Curtius, see Schröder, *Lexikon der hamburgischen Schriftsteller* p. 561. But Curtius's *Exhortatio inclytae rei publicae, cur Judaei a congressu, conversatione et praxi Medicorum arcendi sint* (Hamburg, 1632) is dated after Benedict a Castro's defense. (Friedenwald, *Jews in Medicine* [vol. 1, p. 56], does not seem to notice the problem.)

74. Castro, *Flagellum calumniantium* (prefatory letter): "Quid? Medici non agunt de conscientia, animaeve salute, sed de corporis valetudine, morumque extirpatione, et curatione, et sic medicos Hebraeos non eo quod Hebraei (siquidem non est questio de religione), sed eo quod sint indocti, minimeque medicinam calleant artem reprobare debebat."

75. Ibid., pp. 21–22: "Exempli gratia si interrogavero quare tu monarchiam medicam ambis? dices dubio procul qui Medicus es Christianus, Haec assertio profecta stulta est et nullius momenti. . . ."

76. Ibid., p. 77–78: "Cur Celeberrimi Medici Germani (inter quos primum occupat doctissimus Sennertus) numquam tale argumentum (lacerandi bonos) susceperunt tractandum?"

4

The Medicus-Politicus and the Catholic Context

Jacob Martini's *Apella medicaster bullatus oder Judenarzt* and von Hörnigk's *Medicaster Apella oder Juden Artzt* are one kind of extreme against which to set such physicians as Abraham Zacutus and Rodrigo a Castro. The writers in this anti-Jewish vein sometimes sound shrill, their arguments often seem mere hearsay, and by pointing to the fact that the great physician Sennert, professor at Wittenberg, then still the citadel of Lutheran theology, did not engage in similar polemics, Benedict a Castro effectively suggested that such authors were lightweights in medicine and theology. But there is another extreme that requires our attention, a pole I find most powerfully represented by Girolamo Bardi in his *Medicus politico Catholicus*, a work that takes me close to the end of my time-frame.[1] After a glance at Bardi, I intend to reverse chronology and compare Castro with what before Zacchia was possibly the most quoted book on medical ethics by a Catholic physician—or more precisely by a physician *Catholice sentiens* ("feeling as a Catholic"), as Zacchia likes to put it—namely Battista Codronchi's *De Christiana ac tuta medendi ratione* (1591). There can be no doubt that Codronchi represents more centrally Roman Catholic positions than Bardi. We will study an instructive case from his praxis (showing the physician butting against the limits of his discipline) and try to determine the reason why Castro is silent about the work by Codronchi most closely relating to his *Medicus-Politicus*.

The Physician-Priest: Bardi's Medicus politico Catholicus

It is no accident that I have no factual proof (other than possibly the title of his work) that Bardi is writing against Rodrigo a Castro's *Medicus-Politicus*, for Bardi says that he is deliberately keeping silent about his spiritual adversaries (p. 562), an omission that unquestionably adds urbanity and perhaps even persuasiveness to his book. Bardi also takes me to another boundary of my interest by his iatrochemical leanings; but while these inclinations are evident and are possibly even relevant to his central argument, as I will suggest later, Bardi by his frequent drawing on support from Hippocrates and Galen (and his admiration for such a physician as Antonio Ponce de Santacruz [p. 160]) still essentially presents himself as a "rational," not a Paracelsian physician, and therefore deserves a place in this study.

Born in Rapallo in 1603, Bardi studied for six years with the Jesuits, until ill health induced him to leave the Society. As "magister extraordinarius philosophiae," he taught both Aristotle and Plato for several years at Pisa, but unquestionably inclined toward Plato and Ficino, whom he called the "Platonic phoenix" (*fenice platonica*); such Platonic bias would seem quite appropriate at Pisa, which is, after all, the university of Florence, although Charles B. Schmitt has taught us to distrust such generalizations.[2] Ultimately Bardi attained doctorates in medicine and in theology and (by a dispensation of Pope Alexander VII) was allowed to practice medicine. He died in 1667 in Rome. His book *Medicus politico Catholicus* presents the thesis that a *nexus harmonicus* (p. 205) between theology and medicine is "most noble" (*nobilissimus*) or desirable.

In typical Renaissance fashion, the link is argued both historically and synchronically. In ancient history, Bardi reports in the chapter entitled "Physician-Priests" (*De sacerdotibus medicis*), it was the priests who judged cases of leprosy (p. 197), and he carries his argument one notch further by giving a list of clerics who wrote on medicine. People who think that medicine was invented by man err, for medicine was ultimately created by God: "Since the Most High created medicine as necessary for humankind, its origin should not be traced back to other hands than divine ones without insult not only to medicine itself but to its Creator."[3] Of course the divine origin of medicine is to some extent a commonplace in the Judeo-Christian tradition; even Rodrigo a Castro had devoted a brief chapter of his *Medicus-Politicus* to it under the title: "Explanation of the Passage from Ecclesiasticus [38] according to which Medicine is from God."[4] There Castro had made a weak diplomatic bow to those arguing the primacy of the concern for the soul over the care of the body: "To these arguments I briefly reply that in illnesses it is best to appease (*placare*) God first, but then also useful and necessary to use medications."[5] Bardi has a more specific application of his glance at medical history: for him it is a short distance from the hands of the Divine Physician to the medical hands of the divine, i.e. of the cleric.

Of course Bardi knows (not least from personal experience) of the papal injunction forbidding monks and clerics to practice medicine—he refers to it (pp. 203–04)—but he adds (somewhat sophistically, no doubt, since this matter has little to do with the actual practice of medicine) that certainly physicians can always become clerics. His own experience apparently gives him the confidence to announce in the margin (p. 205): "Dispensation is easily obtained for all."

The excursion into the past is Bardi's means of arguing his specific ideal of physicians in the present: "They carry with them a panacea not so much to counter diseases as to eradicate sins by the roots, prepared both for the office of priests and physicians. No wonder that one of them may fling aside his flasks and six-foot long terms."[6] Thus his ideal physicians are "learned men, who practice sacred medicine with holiness and devoutness."[7] Perhaps surprisingly, if we remember that for many earlier theologians Galen represented the tradition of "medical materialism."[8] Bardi even marshals the support of the "Ethnic" Galen for his position, or rather, by a significant shift, for a related one: "Galen makes the treatment of body and mind one" (p. 305, margin). For modern readers, this insistence that the habits of mind (*animi mores*) and the condition of the body (*recta constitutio corporis*) are interdependent, ultimately a tenet basic to humoral medicine, may be Bardi's strongest suit.

The uses, however, to which Bardi puts the advocated bond (*foedus*) between medicine and theology go beyond a holistic approach to illness: by means of that potent union he tries to solve some of the specific problems that were nagging contemporary theologians and physicians. I give but two examples to indicate the direction of his thought: his ideal physicians will be equipped to distinguish between "uterine furor" (thought to be merely physical) from that fury caused by the devil "by which in Perugia the Blessed Angela of the Fransiscan Order was so strangely ravaged in her genital parts" (p. 347). In particular, Bardi's model physicians will not judge what is divine by the yardstick of the elements of this world, "so that they are not deceived by vain knowledge, of which Jérome Monteux, the royal French physician, is a striking example, who in his medical works thought that the wounds of Saint Francis, which were divinely imprinted, should be explained by a lofty imagination."[9]

Since Bardi, as I have said, deliberately does not mention his spiritual adversaries, I have no proof that he was writing against

Rodrigo a Castro. (He mentions Jews only once: in the context of superstitious remedies derived from heretics and Jews [p. 357]). But Castro's work on women's diseases and his *Medicus-Politicus* were of course very well known in Italy, as can be proved by dozens of references to them, for instance in Paolo Zacchia's enyclopedic *Quaestiones medico-legales* (3d ed., 1651). Whether demonstrable reaction to Castro's encompassing book or not, Bardi's attempt to blend medicine and theology is the polar opposite to Castro's aim of separating the two. It is quite possible that Bardi's iatrochemical inclinations, faint as they may have been, confirmed his belief in the nexus or *foedus* between physician and priest/magus/alchemist, for a version of this belief is almost invariably the axiomatic starting point of alchemical writers. In this respect also, Bardi contrasts with Castro, who sharply censured alchemy and alchemists.[10]

Extreme as Bardi's position may seem with his advocacy of a nexus that (if taken literally and personally) requires papal dispensation, his basic stand is not far removed from what is probably the most influential work of Catholic medical ethics of the sixteenth century, or at least the one quoted most often, Battista Codronchi's *De Christiana ac tuta medendi ratione . . . opus piis medicis praecipue, itemque aegrotis, et ministris, atque etiam sacerdotibus ad confitendum admissis utilissimum* (Ferrara, 1591; republished, 1629). Bardi refers to it always with admiration, and since Castro's *Medicus-Politicus* is quite obviously written against it and similar works, I may be allowed to reverse chronology and briefly characterize Codronchi's work.

Codronchi (1547–1628) was born in Imola and, after studying medicine at Bologna, returned there to practice medicine and write. In addition to his book on medical ethics, which does not seem to be a favorite of modern historians of medicine (the recent *Dizionario biográfico degli Italiani* characterizes it as "uno pedante casista di morale professionale"), Codronchi wrote a work on witchcraft published (in 1595) together with a book on forensic medicine (*De methodo testificandi*), which is generally recognized as important. The contradictions in this physician become strikingly apparent when the same dictionary article that characterizes his "radical conservatism in the scientific field" gives him high marks for innovative observation in his book on rabies (*De rabie, hydrophobia communiter dicta*, 1610), in which Codronchi remarked that the disease was transmitted through the poison of infected animals. His treatise on medical ethics, divided into two books with a total of fifty chapters or sections, is about half the length of Castro's. Each section highlights a deontological proposition by discussing the way a physician may "sin" in the practice of medicine. While these chapters follow no particular logical sequence (in a sense they form a checklist for evaluating the behavior of the physician and his assistants), the scale expressing the relative gravity of malpractice is taken almost exclusively from moral theology: "without any sin" (*sine ullo peccato*), "light fault" (*culpa levis*), "serious sinning" (*gravis peccare*), "capital offense" (*delictum capitale*), and sin calling for excommunication (*praeter peccatum excommunicatur*). Codronchi, whose work (according to its frontispiece) was printed with official permission, is deliberately and expressly applying moral-theological standards to the practice of medicine, and his application is sometimes even a touch tautological (as when he says, without referring to a specific instance like euthanasia, that the physician who uses poison to harm or kill someone sins). An exception, i.e. a piece of reasoning that might be distinguished as more properly medical, is the chapter (lib. 1, c. 23) in which he disagrees with the moral theologian and casuist Navarro, who exempted *empirici*, i.e. not academically trained healers and possibly Paracelsians, from having to know exactly how their prescription works—for the proper physician such ignorance would be sinful—and allowed them a limited role in health care. Like most "rational" physicians, Codronchi has no use for *empirici*. Another exception, although more debatably so, is Codronchi's opposition to curing by friction a type of what used to be called "hysteria" or the "suffocation of the mother," a subject that will concern us in the next chapter.

Codronchi's attempt to harmonize the physician's comportment with Church doctrine is pervasive and was of course recognized as his primary intention by contemporaries. The renowned physician Mercuriale wrote him a letter, included as part of the "paratextual" material prefacing the book, praising the author for his "most apt conjunction of the 'dogmas' of physicians and laymen with Christian teachings."[11] Reading the work, Rodrigo a Castro would have been struck no doubt by the section which Codronchi entitled, "A Physican Who Turns to a Jewish Colleague for Consultation in Treatment . . . Sins" (lib. 1, c. 37). To draw a Jewish doctor into a case or to purchase medication from a Jewish pharmacist is here called a mortal sin (*peccatum morte dignum*), a judgment mitigated only by the casuistic escape clause that the absence of a suitable Christian physician may excuse the transgression. To support this warning against Jews, Codronchi draws on the traditional commonplace that "that nation" (*gens illa*) is taught shifts and ruses to harm rather than respect "us" (p. 112), and then adds the relevant papal pronouncements.

Since problems of forensic medicine often closely relate to ethical problems, it may bear on my topic that Codronchi also wrote a book entitled *The Method of Testifying* (*Methodus testificandi*),[12] the first chapter of which, incidentally, includes a discussion of detecting those who simulate diseases. Castro, who to my knowledge does not refer to Codronchi's book on medical ethics, refers to this work in his chapter on the same subject, the physician's testifying in court.[13] Although a detailed comparison between their views would be interesting, it would lead me beyond my topic. Instead, and particularly since I want to give some impression of how this programmatic harmonizer, so articulate on a variety of ethical questions, proceeded in practice, I would like to quote the most personal account of a medical case of Codronchi's that I have found. It is from his book *Diseases by Witchcraft and Witches* and leads me to a topic I have touched on repeatedly already, namely to describe the way Renaissance physicians resolved problems at the margin of what they considered their competence.

Renaissance Physicians and the Moral-Theological "Expert"

In *Diseases by Witchcraft and Witches* (1st ed., 1595), Codronchi writes:

> A few years ago, my daughter Francesca, then ten months old and in the charge of a nurse, suddenly lost an inordinate amount of weight and more and more often heaved heavy sighs. She cried constantly when being changed and acted ill beyond the habit of children who, however much they experience discomfort or pain, will usually quiet down when being unwrapped and have some respite. Finding no influence of a "praeternatural" [meaning here "pathological"] condition and also after changing the nurse, my wife, as the child got worse, became suspicious that, since the girl was unusually pretty, she had been put under a spell by some old hag out of hate or envy. When she therefore searched the bed, she indeed found signs of witchcraft, namely peas, grains of coriander, a piece of coal and a chip of the bone of a deceased person, some compact matter I could not make out, which an experienced exorcist (*quidam peritus exorcista*) reported to be the kind made with menstrous blood by wicked women. In addition there were some feathers

joined skilfully by threads so that they could easily be put on a cap as is the fashion. After all this had been burned in holy fire (*omnibus igne benedicto combustis*) and after three days of exorcisms and other holy remedies, she began to improve and gain weight, so that we would have thought her cured. However, a few days later, when she was again restless and cried a lot, another search of the same bed revealed some further instruments. After these had been burned, her health seemed to be restored. Yet in the full moon of the month, after she had spent a whole night crying and without sleep, she turned ash color in the morning and her face changed so drastically from what it had been the evening before that it was both a pitiful and unusual thing to see. A new search of the bed revealed two little pieces of a dry nut and of white bone, nine or ten fish bones, shaped in the likeness of combs with which little crowns were very skillfully shaped from various objects. When these had been delivered to the fire and after a change of location as well as after application of all the other and more valid helps by an experienced exorcist, she recovered with God's blessing and without any natural remedy. Thus it seems that God has allowed spells, as I experienced in my daughter, something that I had given little credit in others. In order to know such illnesses and their cure, I began to look for books of that persuasion and to read them and give them trust. Having learned from them and from the experienced exorcist a great deal and also from observing many patients, I feel that I took on that labor willingly in order to help others. Among the authors whom I happened to read was Claudius Gulliaudus, a most learned interpreter of Holy Scripture, who, interpreting St. Paul's epistle to the Galatians, on the subject of witchcraft accurately describes my daughter's illness, which according to him is called *le mal de Vauldorzerie* by some and from which children languish, lose weight, toss about in pain, and sometimes yell and cry incessantly. I have observed all these symptoms and signs in my daughter.[14]

At first sight Codronchi's account may seem commonplace for the period: it agrees with many others on the subject of spells. It appears to differ from the kind of report that fills the pages of the *Malleus maleficarum* only by the fact that the *venefica*, the witch, is not named—in fact, by a relative lack of interest in discovering the perpe-trator of the spell. At the same time, it reveals much about Codronchi: it is not only the most personal text I have found in his writings (as I indicated above), but, though not placed at the beginning of his book *Diseases by Witchcraft*, it represents, as it were, its existential beginning of the entire book.

While this pivotal function of the report can hardly be denied, one may with some justification question its relevance to medical eth-ics, for Codronchi shows no clear indication of a moral dilemma, but seems to proceed along a path that seems natural or at least proper to him—roughly the way any Catholic was supposed to proceed in such circumstances. After Codronchi's wife becomes suspicious that the daughter's illness has no "preternatural causes" (these would include injury or poison; "natural causes" would point to the internal compo-sition of the body, "non-natural" to climate and diet), but what in the period would usually have been called "hyper-physical" ones, a search is made. The suspicious and indefinable objects found under the mattress are presented to an "experienced exorcist," in the Italian context of course a priest, for inspection and analysis. What follows is an elaborate three-day ritual involving "holy fire" and other exor-cisms as well as more "holy remedies," almost certainly including fast and prayer and possibly also contrition and Communion. This proce-dure is repeated at least once, most likely twice ("application of all the other and more valid helps"), again as directed by the "experi-enced exorcist" (*exorcista peritus*). At the same time, because of the eti-ology of the disease, the physician withholds any "natural remedy" until his young daughter recovers.

But the story does not end there. The experience turns the physi-cian from a skeptic into a believer in witchcraft and thus is a kind of conversion story, with a 'before' and 'after' characteristic of the genre. Therefore it may not be insignificant that Codronchi reports that his wife had the first suspicions, although we have no indication of a mar-ital dispute about how to proceed with the troublesome illness. The experience stimulated his theoretical and practical interest in diseases by magical spells: he learns from the expert exorcist, from books by experts (he singles out an exegete of Scripture, i.e. a theologian), and from his own observation. In a limited way he himself thus becomes an expert. His expertise remains medical, essentially a knowledge of when to withhold medical services and rely on the expert member of the clergy.

Codronchi does not tell us whether he would himself use incantations in therapy or participate in them. Several decades later, this is the primary point of contention for Paolo Zacchia in this matter when he says: "All the difficulty is with the incantations."[15] Zacchia points out that "most of the ancients" not only do not allow them, but mock at them. But then he has to concede that some ancients (including Galen) and many moderns allow them. As a Roman Catholic writing in Rome, he has to point out in particular that popes and authorities on canon law accept them. Finally, in a grammatically most interesting construction, he expresses his personal opinion while at the same time unsaying it: "But beyond them [the authorities just named] very many authorities of Holy Scripture give them [the incantations] more than modest trust so that I, who otherwise have no faith in such matters, would not dare simply to deny incantations."[16] The "I would not dare," no doubt part of a special code adopted in a period of strict licensing, effectively sets off the physician's opinion from that of the theological authorities.

By comparison, Rodrigo a Castro, who is not subject to this type of restriction (though of course not free from a variety of other pressures), can afford to speak differently on spells and charms. Tellingly, he begins a section on spells (*Medicus-Politicus*, bk. 5: "De fascinatione") with a programmatic rejection: *rejecimus* (we rejected). His discussion of the phenomenon called "evil eye" sets the stage for the method he will adopt throughout to disparage reports of spells. "Nothing is more frequent than that," he says, "in the mouth of the common people (*vulgares*) and mostly women" (p. 205). Magic is primarily a matter of ignorant women: it is "female trifling" (*nugacitas muliebris*, p. 206) or "figments of little women" (*anicularum figmenta*, p. 205), and his rendering of strange happenings is permeated by an array of distancing verbs of reporting, claiming, saying, etc. (*dicunt, afferunt, contendunt, creduntur*), all of which withhold the author's belief. If old women are charged with doing harm, it is not, according to him, the influence of menstrous blood, as was widely believed, for menstrous blood, while being *vituosus* (harmful, bad), is not poisonous (p. 211). The modern reader would be ill advised to dismiss this as a pseudodistinction, only revealing once again Castro's misogynist tendencies. For this is precisely the kind of discourse that to his readers marks him out as an expert, not in theology of course, but in medicine. Finally he even comes up with a natural explanation of how presumed witches exert influence on children: "The ugly appearance of some old hags by their ill-shaped foulness could so thoroughly terrify young children and fear of them could so stir up their humors that a disease to which a delicate body was already disposed could break out sooner."[17] The physical account of the phenomenon, which hedges all the Aristotelian or scholastic bets by making the old hags apparently accidental rather than efficient causes of disease, keeps it firmly within the purview of the physician's expertise.

Codronchi had seemingly lived in a different world. From its very first sentence (in the "Epistola nuncupatoria"), Codronchi's work on medical ethics, *De Christiana ac tuta medendi ratione*, had emphasized the bond (*coniunctio*) between body and soul and particularly the reciprocal influence of moral habits and physical health. Conceding that medical cure was said to start from the body and proceed to the soul while the (moral) theologian's approach started from the soul to influence the body, his point had been that the aim of both was really one. This unity of enterprise served him as justification for writing the work in hand, and by the same conjunction or unity he defended himself against the charge of "arrogance" that he felt might be leveled by potential critics against a physician weighing and determining the gravity of sin of others, i.e. venturing into the field of the moral theologian. (He thought that his readers would prefer assimilating such matter from a physician.)

My point is that what speaks through Codronchi's book is not some isolated bias against this or that group of physicians or this or that medical procedure, but that his entire endeavor is of a piece with convictions he thinks firmly grounded in Christian orthodoxy. Chapter 37 of book one (on the question whether Jewish physicians may be consulted) is not a momentary lapse into anti-Jewish prejudice (with reference to ruses [*doli*] to which Jews are said to be given and to an unnamed Jewish physician who "who once killed some Emperor by poison"[18]), but integrated in the purpose of the work, which is to show that physicians and Christian theologians work hand-in-hand at the same enterprise. While the topic of how enemies ought to be treated by physicians is not discussed, it would have seemed to a reader like Rodrigo a Castro that Jews were indeed considered spiritual enemies. Close adherence to what was advocated by Codronchi would have made it impossible for Castro to practice medicine.

No wonder, then, that Castro made a fresh start to think through the aims and liabilities of the physician's work, a project "scarcely yet attempted" (as he put it), and culminating twenty-three years after

De Christiana medendi ratione in his *Medicus-Politicus*. We may surmise that writing the work would have deeply involved him, although later (in a complimentary letter printed in Zacuto's *Praxis*) he referred to it, no doubt by a *topos modestiae*, as a "pastime" or "trifle" of his old age (*lusus senectutis*). No wonder also that he did not mention Codronchi's then best-known and most often cited work (although he referred to Codronchi's book on the physician's testifying in court). We surmised earlier that Castro reacted strongly to Henriques' position on lying, so extreme and rigorist, possibly because Henriques, another Lusitanus, did not want to be implicated with New Christians and Marranos. In that case also, Castro failed to identify the person who most likely triggered his radical rethinking of the subject, medical pretense or ruse. (We noticed that Castro had been trained at the same university by some of the same professors.)

While Castro's *Medicus-Politicus* is a well-organized treatise, Codronchi's book on the Christian physician, divided into two books of very unequal length (43 and 7 chapters respectively), is essentially a list of situations in which a physician might lapse into various degrees of culpability. The break between books one and two seems quite arbitrary, and so is the order of the various problems or "chapters." More "books" could easily be added or the second book could be integrated with the first without much changing the nature of the work: a handy reference with astute discussions of situations for which Codronchi thought a Christian physician's moral sensitivity ought to be raised.

To note the difference of intellectual aims is not to disparage Codronchi's book, so often adduced in Zacchia's later account of ethical (he said "medico-legal") problems in medicine. In the next chapter, we will return to one of the ethical issues to which Codronchi devotes an entire chapter (bk. 1, chap. 21), moral scruples about the cure for the condition called "suffocation of the mother." Arcane as the issue may appear to the modern reader, the notoriety it was soon to acquire after Codronchi (apparently the first physician to discuss it in detail) picked it up, showed that he had his finger on the pulse of the time.

NOTES

1. Girolamo Bardi, *Medicus politico Catholicus, seu medicinae sacrae tum cognoscendae, tum faciundae idea* (Genoa, 1644).

2. See *Dizionario biográfico degli Italiani* (Rome: 1960–). The entry on Bardi by C. Colombero mentions that he attended the medical lectures by "Rodrigo De Castro." This physician, sometimes catalogued under the name Rodrigues, should not be confused with the author publishing in Hamburg. Schmitt says (on the sixteenth century): "Far too much stress has been laid on the distinction between 'Paduan Aristotelianism' and 'Florentine Platonism'" ("Philosophy and Science in Sixteenth-Century Italian Universities," in *The Aristotelian Tradition and Renaissance Universities* [London: Variorum Reprints, 1984]: item XV, p. 299).

3. Bardi, *Medicus Politico Catholicus*, p. 324: "Cum medicinam Altissimus creaverit tanquam humano generi necessariam, nec ad alias manus, quam divinas, eius ortus referri debeat, sine iniuria non tam ipsius Medicinae, quam Dei ipsius Creatoris."

4. *Medicus Politicus*, lib. 1, c. 9: "Medicinam a Deo esse, explicatur locus Ecclesiastici."

5. Ibid., p. 31: "His breviter appunctis, respondeo, in morbis optimum esse, Deum prius placare, deinde etiam utile et necessarium medicamentis uti."

6. Bardi, *Medicus Politico Catholicus*, p. 270: "Panaceam non tam ad morbos expugnandos secum ferunt, sed ad extirpanda radicitus, in utrumque parati Sacerdotum functi officio, et Medicorum. Mirum si ex his unus projicit ampullas, et sexquipedalia verba."

7. Ibid., p. 271: "viri Docti, qui Medicinam sacram sancte, pieteque faciunt." Darrel W. Amundsen has written lucidly on the complexities of legal pronouncements governing the clergy's practicing medicine; see "Medieval Canon Law on Medical and Surgical Practice by the Clergy," *Bulletin of the History of Medicine* 52 (1978): 22–144.

8. See Owsei Temkin, *Galenism: Rise and Decline of a Medical Philosophy* (Ithaca: N.Y., and New York: Cornell University Press, 1973), p. 88.

9. Bardi, *Medicus Politico Catholicus*, p. 348: ". . . ne eos decipiat inanis philosophia, quemadmodum magna temeritate factum est a Hieronymo Montuo Gallo Regio Medico, qui in opusculis Medicis putavit vulnera D. Francisci divinitus impressa, in altiorem imaginationem fuisse referenda."

10. See *Medicus-Politicus*, lib. 1, c. 6, entitled, "Explicatur atque rejicitur chymicorum secta."

11. Mercuriale in Codronchi, *De Christiana medendi ratione*: ". . . aptissima medicorum ac profanorum dogmatum cum Christianis praeceptis coniunctio. . ."

12. This work is added to his book *De vitiis vocis* (Frankfurt, 1597).

13. *Medicus-Politicus*, lib. 4, c. 11 (p. 258).

14. Codronchi, *De mobis veneficis, et veneficiis libri IV* (Milan, 1618; 1st ed., 1595), pp. 43–44: "Annis n. superioribus Francesca filia mea decem menses nacta, apud nutricem insigni macie est affecta, saepe, ac saepius magna suspiria edebat; et quando difasciatur semper plorebat, aegreque ferebat se defasciari praeter puerorum morum, qui quamvis sint male affecti, vel dolore aliqui detenti, cum fasciae solvuntur quiescere, ac delectationem capere tum solent, nulla inventa causa praeter naturali affectus, nutriceque

mutata, cum in deterius laberetur, subiit suspitio uxori meae, cum esset puella admodum venusta invidentiae causa, vel odii cuiusdam vetulae, veneficio esse affectam. Quae propter culcitram inquirens nonnulla signa veneficii reperiit, ciceres nempe, grana coriandrorum, frustum carbonis, et ossis defuncti, rem quandam compactam mihi incognitam, quam fieri ab his improbis foeminis ex quibusdam cum sanguine menstruo mixtis, retulit quidam peritus exorcista; praeterea quasdam plumas ita quibusdam filis artificiose insertas, ut pileo, ut mos est, applicari facile possent; quibus omnibus igne benedicto combustis, et adhibitis per triduum exorcismis et aliis remediis sacris coepit melius habere, et carnem assumere, ita ut curatam existimaremus. Nihilominus transactis nonnullis diebus, cum esset valde inquieta, et multum ploraret, eodem lectulo denuo explorato, inventa sunt nonnulla alia instrumenta, quibus crematis, sanati restitui visa est: Attamen in plenilunio mensis cum plorabunda noctem totam insomnem duxisset, mane colore cinericio fuit affecta, et ita mutata facie ab ea, quae vesperi erat, ut esset res non minus lachrimis, quam admiratione digna: explorato denuo lectulo inventa sunt frustula duo nucis siccae, et ossis albi, novem, vel decem ossa piscium, quae erant fabricata instar pectinum, quibus pectuntur cum quibusdam corollis mira arte ex variis rebus paratis: quibus igni traditis, mutata domo, et omnis aliis, et validioribus per exorcistam peritum adhibitis auxiliis, Dei benedicio absque ullo remedio naturali convaluit: quod quidem veneficium fortasse Deus permisit, ut in mea puella experiter, quod in aliis parum credebam veritatis habere: Pro quorum morborum cognitione, et curatione, coepi quaerere libros huius professione, eosque legere, et illis fidem habere: ex quibus, peritoque exorcistacum multa didicerim, libenter hunc laborem suscepi aliis opitulandi studio, inter alios autem auctores, quos mihi legere contigit, fuit Claudius Gulliaudus interpres sacrarum literarum eruditissimus, qui interpretando Epistolam D. Pauli, quam ad Galata missit, agens de fascino adamussim morbum filiae meae scribit, quem Gallice a quibusdam dici *le mal de Vauldorzerie* ait, et ex quo infantes tabescunt, macrescunt, ac misere torquentur, et aliquando incessanter clamant, et flent; quae omnia symptoma; et signa in filia mea observavi."

15. *Quaestiones medico-legales* (3d ed., Amsterdam, 1651), lib 2, tit. 2, quaestio 13 (p. 87): "Tota difficultas est de Incantationibus." Each book of Zacchia's big work bears the imprimatur.

16. Ibid., p. 88: "Sed praeter haec non modicam fidem faciunt permultae sacrae Scripturae auctoritates, ita ut non ausim ego, qui alias huiusmodi rebus nullam fidem habeo, incantationes simpliciter negare."

17. Rodrigo a Castro, *Medicus Politicus*, p. 211: "Trux aspectus vetularum deformi suo squallore potuit infantulos perterre facere, timor concitare humores, ut citius morbus erumpat, ad quem tenellum corpusculum iam erat dispositum."

18. *De Christiana medendi ratione*, p. 113: ". . . Medicus Iudaeus olim Imperatorem quendam veneno interfecit." A note in the margin refers to the French writer on Roman law André Tiraqueau.

5

The Moral Dilemma about Removing Seed

In choosing to treat ethical issues concerning sexuality for the remaining chapters of this book, I have been influenced by interests of modern historians of literature and of gender. Even within the topic and period boundaries I set myself, it would have been impossible to give a comprehensive survey of medical ethics. Since the need to be selective imposed itself, I chose areas related to the field of gender studies, in which some of the most exciting historical studies are being conducted today. Therefore the remaining chapters will be divided by gender. But consciousness of my own biases also leads me to admit that for many Renaissance physicians, other problems may have been just as pressing as, or even more important than, the moral dilemma of what was called "removing seed." Nevertheless this seems to have been a new and troubling problem, both difficult in itself and difficult to speak about, because it is surrounded by sexual and religious taboos.

"This matter is so difficult in the medicine of our day that nothing else, in my judgment, comes close," says the Spanish physician Juan Rafael Moix (or Moxius) in his book *De methodo medendi per venae sectionem morbos muliebres acutos* (Geneva, 1612), a book ostensibly on venesection, but also treating many peripheral and ethical issues in considerable detail. I cannot exclude the possibility that in the sentence quoted he meant the removal of male as well as female seed, but the context makes clear beyond any doubt that primarily on his mind was the ethical question whether it was licit for physicians to remove the supposed spoilt (Latin *depravatus*) *female* seed from the genitals or genital area. Certainly important contemporaries, among whom were the physicians Cortesi and Zacchia, understood him that way and cited him, agreeing with his evaluation (but not necessarily with his solution to the moral dilemma). These citations also indicate that Moxius's thick book, which now exists in few libraries and (as far as I can tell) always in marginal condition, was important, and that he was not considered an esoteric writer, far out in some postmonastic Iberian field. Since Renaissance physicians argue their solutions to these ethical problems on the basis of considerable physiological detail—Cortesi gives several folio pages of detailed description of the female genital organs plus schematic drawings)—a minimal rehearsal of traditional physiology is in order.

Female Seed and Menses

The "difficult matter" referred to by Moxius is related to, but far from identical with, the controversy about the existence of female seed. In their book *Sexuality and Medicine in the Middle Ages*, Danielle Jacquart and Claude Thomasset report that "the polemic concerning female sperm lasted from beginning to end of the Middle Ages."[1] And just as the Middle Ages did not invent the polemic, so the controversy continued through the Renaissance. Since I am only concerned with ethical problems surrounding the so-called removal of "male and female sperm" from the genitals, I can be brief in the history of the polemic, in which the authority of Aristotle (holding that only males have seed) is opposed to most other ancient physiologists, according to whom women also have some kind of semen. According to the latter, the human fetus is the result of the mixture and interaction of both types of seed. Hippocrates' view that there was female ejaculation was powerful support for the notion of female seed: "The woman also ejaculates from all her body, sometimes in the womb— and the womb becomes moist—sometimes outside if the womb is open wider than should be the case."[2] As he summarizes the controversies raging in his discipline, i.e. medicine, Francisco de Valles (Franciscus Valesius, 1524–1592), in the second half of the sixteenth century, still sees the relationship as an all against one, namely Aristotle; and Valles enthusiastically sides with the overwhelming majority. It may have suited his purpose to omit some modern adherents of Aristotle, who appear in his argument only as "someone" (*aliquis*) and "common philosophers" (*vulgares philosophi*): "But someone may say (for I neglect what is being said by the common philosophers on this subject): If both had semen, both would have power; then the woman could conceive without coition, just by her self. But nothing is more absurd. One needs to reply that female semen, even though it has powers, as we said, yet is of less strength than that it might alone suffice for conception, for it is colder than the male variety."[3] Valles's view influenced Rodrigo a Castro's important book on women's diseases that went through many editions in the seventeenth century—he is cited by Castro in this context.[4]

For Renaissance physicians boldly to attack ancient authority, as they often do, does not by itself indicate that they base their view on observation. In what is possibly the best book on women in the Renaissance, Ian Maclean says correctly: "The situation by the end of the sixteenth century is quite confused, but it may be said with a certain degree of confidence that the general context of medicine remains Galenist, while the work of Aristotle and the 'neoterici' is in dispute, leading to accusations of incompetence and plagiarism."[5] Arcane as it may seem to the modern reader, the notion of female seed in emitted fluids has important implications beyond the limits of my topic: as scholars writing on the subject (for instance Maclean; Jacquart and Thomasset) are aware, the idea of female seed (of relative equality of males and females in this respect) could be, and was, used to support an argument for an equal worth of the sexes, while Aristotle's view that woman was a defective human being, or, at least, an imperfect or incomplete version of the male ("fair defect of nature," as Milton's Adam puts it), lent itself to the opposite opinion.

In spite of the striking impression of similarity between the sexology of the Middle Ages and the Renaissance, there are, as Ian Maclean has pointed out, at least two important differences: Gabriele Fallopio's descriptions of the female organs and the rejection by many 'neoterici' of Galen's notion of the correspondence or comparison of male and female genitalia (the idea that one kind is the inverted shape of the other). I will add a third, possibly more subtle, difference, which has to do with the very subject that will occupy us later: a growing sensitivity to the moral dangers of all concerned in "manipulating" female genitalia. I will have to pass over the first two types of Renaissance innovation except in cases where physiology becomes part of an argument in ethics.

As Ian Maclean points out, Rodrigo a Castro denounces the sixteenth-century collection of medical books on women entitled *Gynaecea* (Basel, 1577) as a mixture of "excellent doctrine and wild speculation, which could easily mislead students of medicine,"[6] but Castro himself does not swerve from the Galenic belief in the existence of female seed, using incidentally, with a light touch, the Genesis passage that was to intrigue Milton as support: "If it may be allowed to adduce pages above all nature in natural speculations, we read in 3

Genesis that it is said of the snake, 'I will place enmity between your seed and the seed of the woman.'"[7] Although the argument is made with urbanity and even a distancing awareness of the limits of cogency in such use of a biblical passage, if the argument is meant to count for anything it has to rely on principles like Melanchthon's, namely that the Old Testament and natural/divine law are congruent. It would serve no purpose further to document the dominant Renaissance belief in female seed, except to insist that modern smugness and ahistorical laments about Renaissance lack of observation are out of place. Physical "evidence" can be a dubious matter indeed. Thus the then well-known physician Luis Mercado (like Rodrigo a Castro, he was born of Jewish parents, but had officially converted to Christianity) argues against Aristotle and supports his belief in the existence of female seed by the evidence of experience: "Apart from that [reason by authority], there is no man so inexperienced in sexual matters that he would not feel during coition his penis moisten with female seed and the woman be warmed by that pouring forth (*profusio*) which even the women themselves experience, since they feel themselves getting moist before reception of the male seed."[8]

It was generally believed that female seed shared with menstrual blood the tendency to corrupt and become noxious if for some reason trapped in the female body, a deterioration borne out, according to Renaissance physicians, by dozens of ancient and modern case histories. The two discharges are also often linked by similar names, for both are called *flores* (flowers) through euphemistic transference, possibly by some folk etymology, from *fluores* (plural of *fluor*, "flux"). Jacques Dubois (or Iacobus Sylvius, 1478–1553), an arch-Galenist and teacher of Vesalius, explains: "There are some who call [the menses] *flores*, for they say that as the flower precedes the fruit, so women do not conceive until these discharges have flowed, as almost all practical physicians affirm."[9] English *flowers*, French *fleurs*, and the archaic German *Blume* seem to be loan translations of *flores*. As to menstrual blood, unfortunately neglected in Maclean's brief account of Renaissance female physiology, there are signs in the period that the medieval vilification of it (as described by Jacquart and Thomasset) is changing.[10] I quoted earlier Rodrigo a Castro's distinction that menstrual blood, while harmful, is not poisonous. But although the great physician Mercuriale misses no opportunity to point out that this blood is nothing but "pure blood in excess," and even cites a report that some Gnostic sect not only sacrificed the menses (*mentrua*) but drank them without harm,[11] change is slow in coming. Late in the period, Abraham Zacuto draws up a long list of medical authors (ancient and modern) believing that menstrual blood is *vitiosus* (harmful) and opposes that impressive catalogue to the rare few who think otherwise—he sides with the majority.[12] Ultimately, however, this dissension among the physicians is of only minor significance for the ethical problems arising from the cure to be explained, for there was near agreement that all these fluids, both "suppressed" menses and retained semen, could deteriorate in the womb and turn so noxious as to equal the strongest poison. For Zacuto, as for many physicians, the uterus was "the cloaca of the entire body, the bilge and receptacle of excrements. The weakness of innate heat in the female sex adds to this by not repelling the causes of decomposition."[13] Indeed the poison is so strong that it can lead to sudden death.[14]

The pathological condition of the uterus, or *hystera*, just described represents, of course, the primary one traditionally called "hysteria," which, since Ilza Veith's book on its history, has received considerable and well-deserved attention. (This includes the recent composite edition, by Michael MacDonald, of some English seventeenth-century tracts.)[15] Unfortunately Veith's account of Renaissance thinking about hysteria and its cure is brief, and her presentation of Edward Jorden's *Brief Discourse of a Disease Called the Suffocation of the Mother* (1603) imbalanced by her questionable thesis that Jorden (1569–1632) is transferring "the seat of all hysterical manifestations from the uterus to the brain," a transfer she celebrates as "a major turning point in the history of hysteria" (p. 123). At the same time she has to admit that "his conversion . . . was not entire. He added to the traditional factors of interrupted menstruation and sexual abstinence the idea that 'the perturbations of the minde are often to blame for this and many other diseases.'" Michael MacDonald has questioned Veith's claim and sees Jorden's intent and significance as arising out of the political and religious context of a case on which he took a stand (see MacDonald's introduction). From my perspective, Jorden's account of female physiology and hysteria seems quite traditional. The margins of the three paragraphs on the two types of peccant fluids (blood and sperm) indicate that he relies on such ancients as Hippocrates and Galen, and among the moderns, on Mercado, twice as often as on anyone else (fol. 17v–20). Finally he reaches for the strongest comparisons available in medical literature to suggest the strength of the poison to which female sperm degenerates: the venom of serpent, scorpion, torpedo [a crampfish or electric ray], and a mad dog (fol. 20). The question then remains why Jorden does not mention one of the most frequently listed cures for such cases since antiquity, a cure which was the subject, according to Moxius's view (with which we started), of lively ethical discussions in his time.

The answer is twofold and simple and brings us back to the concerns of medical ethics, which we seem to have abandoned momentarily. Jorden labors with a self-imposed restriction, evident even as he discusses the etiology of the disease:

> The causes of this disease and of the *symptoms* belonging therunto, have ever been found hard to be described particularly: and especially in a vulgar tongue, I hold it not meete to discourse to[o] freely of such matters, and therefore I doe crave pardon if I do but slenderly overpasse some poynts which might be otherwise more largely stood upon. (Fol. 18)

These are the restrictions about writing of sexual matters in English that made Robert Burton, when writing about sex in his *Anatomy of Melancholy*, switch to Latin for entire paragraphs, then, even in his Latin, use a heavy dosage of the rhetorical figure *praeteritio* (in which the writer states that he is omitting something), and at the end of the Latin passage admiringly cite and adapt Rodrigo a Castro's (Latin) words about stylistic decorum and Castro's intention to write for the learned (medical or lay).[16]

If Jorden feels that he has to veil the presentation of the causes of the disease, his restrictions on articulating cures are double. His selection is controlled by what MacDonald has identified as the occasion of the piece, and therefore cures are not Jorden's focus. More important in my context, any detailed discussion of the therapy traditionally indicated (given the causes he has listed earlier: corruption of blood as the result of retention of the menses and corruption of semen) would be indecorous in the medium Jorden has chosen. Thus the final sentence of his pamphlet represents the ultimate figure of omission, the *non plus ultra* of *praeteritio*, for with it he falls silent: "Other matters of government either in the fit or out of the fit, together with the cure in regard of the internal causes, because they are properly belonging to the Physition, I do purposely omit." Jorden's pamphlet or, more generally, books in the vernacular like Philip Barrough's *Methode of Phisick* (1583 and 1590), whatever purposes they may have served, cannot serve as reliable guides to those marginal but extremely instructive areas where physicians wrestled with definition of their duties and the difficulty of expressing them. Jorden's omission demonstrates the need for us to return to Latin texts if we want to learn anything about the traditional cure of this disease and about the moral unease that cure seems to have elicited.

The Physician's Probing Hand and Shame

A widow, 44, sister of Laurentius Athenarius, pastor of the village called Soechtwouda (my teacher in my youth), a woman living in Alkmaer near the crane, in May of 1546 seriously suffered from the suffocation of the mother (*suffocatio uteri*). When she was taken for dead and was lying unconscious, I was urgently called to her. However, it was a case of suffocation because of retained seed (*suffocatio ex semine retento*). The women present were sprinkling her face with wine and bedaubing her nostrils and temples, believing they could wake her thus from her swoon. But they were only making her worse. . . . Therefore I ordered them to quit their moistening, sprinkling, and rubbing with wine. And in order that she might inhale the stench of some of her own hair burned (since no partridge feathers were at hand [for burning]), I moved it constantly before her nostrils for her to smell. Then I gave her feet a painful rubbing, massaging her hard with salt and vinegar under my palms. For their acidity and sting (according to Gradus [Giovanni Matteo Ferrari da Grado, in the fifteenth century]) forces superfluidities downward and brings [the patient] out of the swoon. We also applied bindings to her hips, now relaxing and now tightening them, for all of this, by inflicting pain, stirs matter downward and prevents the rising upward of vapors. In the meantime, because of the urgency of the situation, we asked a midwife to come and apply the following ointment to the patient's genitals, rubbing them inside with her finger. [The recipe for the ointment is given.] And thus she was against hope brought back to consciousness. For such titillation with the finger is commended by all physicians, including Galen and Avicenna, particularly for widows and persons abstaining like nuns, according to Gradus—less so for younger and servant women or those who have a husband; for them a better remedy is to sleep with a man. However, I am of the opinion that this should only be done in very urgent circumstances after other remedies have failed.[17]

PETRI FORESTI
ALCMARIANI
OBSERVATIONVM,
ET CVRATIONVM
MEDICINALIVM
Libær vigefimus-octauus,

DE MVLIERVM MORBIS.

Vnà cum SCHOLIIS.

Ex Officinâ Plantinianâ,
APVD CHRISTOPHORVM RAPHELENGIVM,
Academiæ Lugduno-Bat.Typographum.
CIɔ. Iɔ. IC.

Figure 5.1. Frontispiece of colume 28 of Peter Foreest, *Observationum et curationum medicinalium libri*, Lugdunum Batavorum, 1599 (National Library of Medicine).

The report is by the Dutch physician Peter Foreest (1522–1597), whose medical cases with commentaries (*scholia*) called *observationes* were about the best known such collections about 1600. In the early seventeenth century, almost any medical author in Central Europe, particularly also physicians writing on women's diseases (including Edward Jorden and Hermann Corbeius),[18] would of course have checked Foreest's collection and referred to it. The quoted report is from a section entitled "A Widow's Case of the Suffocation of the Mother Caused by Retained Seed." I have omitted Foreest's detailed reasoning why the attempts of the women (*mulierculae*, literally "little women," always seems pejorative) to revive the patient through sprinkling with aromatica was doomed to failure. In rendering the entirely commonplace theory (not explained by Ilza Veith), Foreest here relies on Rhasis's translator and commentator Gradus, who had explained at length the traditional notion that upward-moving vapors of the womb, sometimes called "the wandering womb," can only be forced back (i.e. down) by ill-smelling odors applied to the nostrils. Therefore the "little women's" perfumes applied to the face would have the undesired effect of exerting an even stronger pull upward.[19]

Foreest's case history consists of three parts: the well-intended but ill-informed attempts by the *mulierculae* (and an explanation of why they are wrong), the various attempts to revive the patient after the physician's arrival, and (with the call for the midwife) the application of the remedy that is effective. The first two parts articulate neatly in sequential narrative form the subject of such discursive accounts as Grado's, but at the same time the second segment does more, for it demonstrates what the physician is advocating: that all other means need to be exhausted and the patient's condition be judged critical before the last remedy is applied. Although Foreest is more emphatic in his call for the midwife, Grado also had a midwife execute the manipulation, and it follows that Grado admits that on the subject of pessaries matrons and midwives (*matrones et obstetrices*) are more experienced than physicians (fol. 457v). Since Foreest relies on the midwife as informant, his diagnostic experience is literally secondhand: we learn that another and similar case is diagnosed as *uterus retractus* (a retracted or "wandering" womb) on the authority of the midwife's report (*sic obstretice dicente*, p. 128).

Because of the shame the physician's probing hand would cause, it is ruled out as improper, just as is deliberately prurient titillation by the midwife. Foreest makes this clear in an aside reporting the objectionable procedure by a colleague (unless the *chirurgus* was of lower status, the medical equivalent of a *muliercula*):

Shameless is also the advice of some woman (*muliercula*) that the patient's pubic hair be pinched to make the hysteric women (*suffocata*) come to themselves. For that was done by a surgeon in a highly shameless manner when his maidservant, who had suddenly collapsed and was lying unconscious, with many people standing about in her bedroom, as I saw. Stirred up by shame, she walked away healed, to the laughter of those present.[20]

It is possible that this pulling and pinching of pubic hair relates to an ancient practice that was already criticized by Soranus and Galen as crudely violent, as Veith reports (p. 115), in which case Foreest's critique might be derivative. But his emphasis is not on violence, but on erotic shame and on violating the patient's deepest sense of privacy. For that reason the case may be close in spirit to Edward Jorden's story reported four years later (1603). In terms of professional ethics and status, it may be significant that Jorden's report also contrasts the gentler ways of a physician with the crudeness of a surgeon:

A yong Maiden also upon some passion of the minde, as it was credibly reported, fell into the fits of the Mother, and being in one of them, a Physitian then present modestly put his hand under her cloathes to feele a windie tumor which shee then had in her backe. But a Surgeon there also present not contented with that manner of examination, offered to take up her cloathes, and to see it bare: wherupon the Maid being greatly offended, took such indignation at it, as it put her presently out of her fit. (Fol. 25–25v)

What Veith says about this hysterical maiden may also hold for the maidservant in Foreest, namely that there is a recognition that another perturbance helps to get the patient out of her hysterical paroxysm (Veith, p. 124). But although Jorden's point expressedly is that "the cause of these affections" can sometimes be removed "by introducing other perturbations of diverse nature" (fol. 25), he is also implying that the surgeon acted indecorously, and is almost as far from advocating such violation in the interest of cure as is Foreest. In terms of Renaissance medical ethics, the point of both medical cases is to suggest that this can be done, but it should not.

The Controversy about Removing Female Seed

As so often in Renaissance medical controversy, the ancients are either expressed or silent partners in the discussion, and before I outline what is perhaps the most striking part of the controversy, Cortesi's disagreement with Moxius, it may be useful to look at one of the *loci classici* most often evoked for this subject matter. My impression that this is indeed the particular medical case whose terms reverberate whenever the removal of female seed is discussed (and such discussion is standard in Renaissance disquisitions on women's diseases) is confirmed by Abraham Zacuto, who devotes several folio pages to four cases involving removal of seed, of which the following (quoted from Galen, *De locis affectis*, 6) is the first:

> I encountered the following story of a woman who had been a widow for a long time. Besides some other disturbances, she was afflicted with nervous tension. When a midwife told her that her womb was pulled up, she thought she should employ remedies customarily used for this ailment. On application the heat of this medicine and the contact with her sexual organs provoked [uterine] contractions associated with the pain and pleasure similar to that experienced during intercourse. As result the woman secreted a large quantity of semen and thus lost the bothersome complaints.[21]

The words "pain and pleasure" (*cum labore et voluptate*) from the action mimicking coition in this celebrated case reverberate through Renaissance medical discussion. Zacuto, who quotes this passage at length, does not engage Galen in an open controversy, but he gives a detailed explanation of how sexual activity weakens the body. The implied comment on the Galenic passage appears to be a warning against sexual activity (of whatever kind) as a remedy. Nevertheless, since he accepts the view that indeed terrible symptoms may arise from retained female semen, he emphasizes the use of drugs that, in terms of humoral medicine, cool and dry the body, thus presumably reducing the production of sperm and allaying sexual desire. The list includes cannabis seeds, but also simples whose powers appear to reside at least in part in their name or shape: agnus castus (the chaste tree; Gr. *agnos* = L. *castus*), *nymphaea* (water lily), and *radix asparagi* (root of asparagus).[22] Although Zacuto is thus not directly addressing the ethical issue of this cure of hysteria his selection of brief texts that he considered important recognized the notoriety of the Galenic passage and once more (and possibly for one of the last times before the passing of the notion of female semen) made it a focus of attention. In his other major work, *De praxi medica* (1634), Zacuto more precisely asks the question, "whether the God-fearing physician is allowed to expel from the uterus the poisonous semen by titillation and friction of the genital area of women in mortal danger, deprived of all their senses and their breathing."[23] But he gives no answer of his own, except by referring to the discussion of others, particularly the "eloquent" Moxius. We also note that the Jewish Lusitanus, expatriate (practicing in Holland), replaces the notion of the Christian physician, promoted by Codronchi's book on medical ethics, by that of the *medicus timens Deum*, "the God-fearing physician."

The caution, of which Zacuto's indirectness and silence is evidence, had been encoded more deliberately by Rodrigo a Castro (on whose book on women's diseases Zacuto often relies) in a parenthetical conditional clause: "Then (if this can be done without crime), the midwife may rub the neck of the uterus with her fingers . . . so that so stimulated the gross humor remaining fixed in the uterus is provoked, warmed up, and excreted."[24] In terms of the contrast pointed out earlier between Castro and Codronchi as authors of Renaissance books on medical ethics, Castro's choice of words here, *sine scelere* (without crime) rather than *sine peccato* (without sin), is significant, since "crime" transfers the possibility of misdeed out of the religious coordinates into secular or civic ones.

In his own commentary or *scholium*, intended to highlight key notions of his treatise for the medical specialist (as he explains in his preface to Part 2), Castro elucidates specifically this conditional clause *si id fieri liceat* (if that can be done [without crime]): "Whether one should by friction applied to the pudendum have the semen flow forth, I leave to the wise [*sapientes*] to discuss, but I note that the semen excreted at that time is not able to generate any more, but is a poisonous and useless excrement of the body and the cause of many ills, often even of death, and, moreover, excreted against the will of the women or at least without their consent."[25] Thus the question of moral defensibility of the procedure is left to "the wise," not to the theologians, as it is usually phrased in that period in Catholic countries when physicians bow out of an ethical question. The substitution may be another element of de-theologizing or laicization of ethical issues that we have observed in Castro elsewhere. In addition, if *meiosis* (making oneself small) is at the core of irony, there may be also a touch of that, since the speaker excludes himself from the wise, possibly suggesting that the matters these wise men resolve are perhaps not so important and therefore they are not so truly wise. At the same time, by explaining that the female patients shed the corrupted seed "against their will or at least without their consent," the expatriate Jewish Lusitanus reveals that he has assimilated thoroughly the distinctions of Iberian moral casuists, for it was one's consent (an act of will) to some sexual fantasy, image, or act that in doubtful circumstances determined whether it was sinful or not.

We may gain a clearer understanding of how the ethical scruple about digital stimulation developed (and that the unambiguous expression of this scruple is a late phenomenon in Renaissance medicine) if we look at the two well-known sixteenth-century collections of gynecological works assembled by Kaspar Wolf (Basel, 1566) and by Israel Spach (Strassburg, 1597, first ed. 1586–88). In the former, where the work *De mensibus mulierum* by Jacques Dubois (the "arch-Galenist of Paris") still mentions titillation without comment, as a means by which *labore et voluptate quasi per coitum* the peccant semen is expelled, there is no evidence that the procedure is questioned or questionable.[26] In the latter, an updated version of the former, i.e. a collection of nineteen famous ancient and modern gynecological authors assembled more than a generation later by Spach (1560–1610) and Bauhin (1560–1624), the same work by Dubois mentioning titillation for evacuation is again present, and the topic is also mentioned without critical comment in the works by Albertino Bottoni (early sixteenth century–1596) and Mercuriale, in both cases with reference to the Galenic passage we cited.[27] But the work by Luis Mercado, *De mulierum affectionibus libri quatuor*, the second longest and arguably the most important work in Spach's collection, shows the beginning of a different sensibility and sensitivity. On the subject of uterine corrupted seed, the famous Spanish writer, personal physician of both Philip II and Philip III, warns: "But one should abstain from titillations which many [authors] recommend for the genitals, even if we see that by that means women are relieved by the excretion of the semen; for we know that the Christian physician is not permitted to do this."[28] The objection by the New Christian Mercado, whose Roman Catholic orthodoxy is sometimes affirmed in prefaces to his books by writers pointing out that some of the physician's children embraced the religious life, is the first time I have found the procedure opposed by a medical doctor.

Before discussing the specific theological and medical objections that became the focus of a lively debate about 1600, we may glance ahead to a passage by the famous French physician François Ranchin, after 1612 chancellor at Montpellier, in order to gauge the change in ethical thinking on this matter from, let us say, the time of the first of the two gynecological compendia mentioned above through the first quarter of the seventeenth century. Ranchin, unquestionably one of the most insightful Roman Catholic physicians of his time—whom I have adduced for that reason in my chapter on pretense in curing— writes on our subject in his *Tractatus de morbis virginum*:

> Very serious and extremely important is the difficulty mentioned, namely whether one is allowed to rub women or handle their parts in their hysterical paroxism. Those who approve do not lack authorities and arguments. First Galen puts forth the story of some widow restored to health by a midwife inserting her finger in her womb and thus evacuating her semen. From this grew the practice that most [women] use instruments skillfully hollowed out and similar in form to the male penis in order to provoke voluntary pollution and guard against hysterical symptoms. Secondly, Avicenna recommends that midwives insert a finger into the vulva and rub it diligently until the seminal material is expelled.[29]

Ranchin then briefly summarizes the physiology that, according to the proponents of the procedure, is supposed to make it work,

> from which it appears that such friction is applied instead of sexual activity (*veneris vicem*) and is a well proven therapy; and therefore they conclude it is inhuman to recommend against the use of that salutary remedy. We, however, following the teaching of the theologians, hold friction of this kind to be abominable and damnable, particularly in virgins, since such pollution may spoil virginity.[30]

If the reader of this study should have difficulty recognizing the Ranchin who, as we saw in the chapter on pretense in curing, was interested in separating the province of the theologian from that of the physician, there is at least a hint of the same preoccupation in the sentence with which Ranchin concludes the discussion of this topic:

"But as far as women (*mulieres*) are concerned, we leave the use of that remedy to their conscience, since it does not behoove Christian physicians to give advice and counsel concerning divine precept."[31]

Ranchin is important as a Catholic physician extraordinarily sensitive to ethical questions and, as his approach to this gynecological dilemma confirms, consistently interested in resolving territorial disputes between physician and theologian. Moral casuists of the period would no doubt have noticed that his particular solution about *mulieres*, and perhaps even that about *virgines* comes dangerously close to a form of indirect influence that (as we shall see in chapter 6) was expressly proscribed: "As a physician, I know that this remedy works, but I cannot recommend it." But for the controversy about the removal of female seed Ranchin's opinion and solution do not seem to have been particularly important: in fact, I cite him merely as an index to show how far medical opinion had swung by the end of the first quarter of the seventeenth century. The most important discussion of the issue, i.e. both the most detailed and the most often referred to in the period, is that of the Spanish physician Moxius, with whose evaluation of its popularity in the medicine of his time we started this chapter. To it we must now turn.

Moxius (or Moix, *fl.* 1587–1612) was born in Gerona and studied at Valencia, where he also practiced medicine. The relevant section (chap. 27) of his book is entitled: "Is the Physician Permitted to Expel Directly the Corrupt Semen that Induces Death?" After explaining the medical side of the problem, Moxius halts and comments: "This is a very difficult and arduous problem that has by now tortured the minds of many."[32] Physicians agree, he reports, that hysteria can indeed be lethal and that of its two causes (retained menses and retained semen), the latter is considered more dangerous. Although Moxius does not mention it, this evaluation goes back to a comment by Galen that precedes his case of the widow considered above.[33] Moxius then reviews that very case, taking particular note of the words *cum labore et voluptate* with which the expelling of the semen is described by Galen. Here he halts again to comment: "This matter is so difficult in contemporary medicine that nothing else, in my judgment, comes close, because all theologians agree that while there may be also healthy semen present, only the peccant part may be expelled directly with any justification."[34] Since he finds the matter highly ambiguous, Moxius takes the reader through both sides of the argument and finally is guided, in the manner of the moral casuists, when

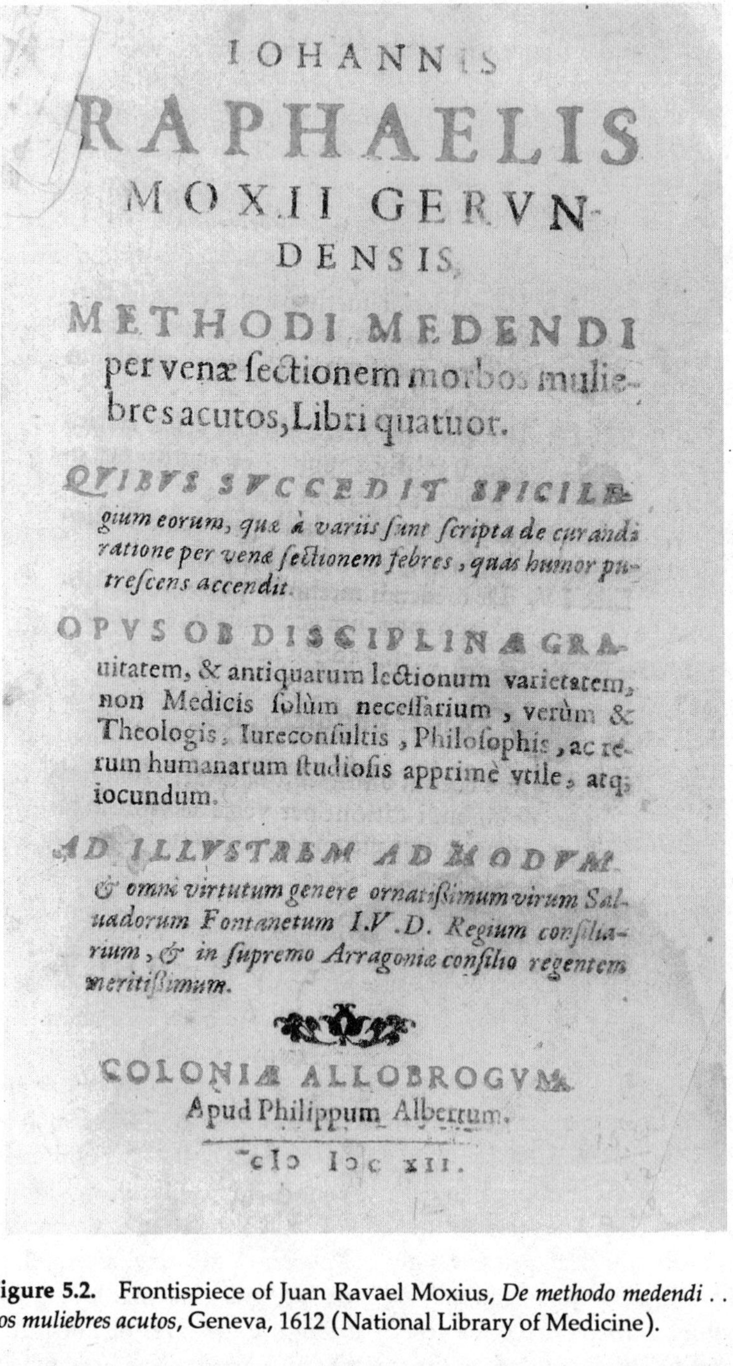

IOHANNIS

RAPHAELIS

MOXII GERVN-
DENSIS,

METHODI MEDENDI
per venæ fectionem morbos muliebres acutos, Libri quatuor.

*QVIBVS SVCCEDIT SPICILE-
gium eorum, quæ à variis funt fcripta de curandà
ratione per venæ fectionem febres, quas humor pu-
trefcens accendit.*

OPVS OB DISCIPLINÆ GRA-
uitatem, & antiquarum lectionum varietatem,
non Medicis folùm neceffarium, verùm &
Theologis, Iureconfultis, Philofophis, ac rerum humanarum ftudiofis apprimè vtile, atq;
iocundum.

*AD ILLVSTREM ADMODVM
& omni virtutum genere ornatiffimum virum Sal-
uadorum Fontanetum I.V.D. Regium confilia-
rium, & in fupremo Arragoniæ confilio regentem
meritiffimum.*

COLONIÆ ALLOBROGVM.
Apud Philippum Albertum.

⌐IↃ IↃC XII.

Figure 5.2.   Frontispiece of Juan Ravael Moxius, *De methodo medendi . . . morbos muliebres acutos*, Geneva, 1612 (National Library of Medicine).

opposing arguments stand in equal balance, by opting for what is "safer" (*tutius*). If one is allowed to abort a dead fetus, he reasons first, should it not be licit to expel this poisonous seed useless for generation, considering that the woman is partially senseless and hardly breathing? He notices that the moral casuist Thomas Sanchez was of that opinion for several reasons that are not foolish (*nec anilis*) at all. In fact he paraphrases Sanchez to say that one should not worry whether good semen is being discharged beyond the original intent of the cure, for the action is necessary for health.[35] According to this argument, one should be permitted to avail oneself of the remedies of nature for expelling harmful substances, even if by accident pollution follows. Finally Moxius quotes Sanchez as arguing that since "all people were permitted to scratch their private parts to relieve some itching, so they were allowed to show what is private to surgeons so that they would heal illnesses, open the parts closed, although pollution could result from that beyond intention."[36] But then Moxius moves to the opposing side, distancing himself from the permissive Sanchez, whom he respects as an earnest theologian. "The opposite and safer view is held by most and without doubt the most earnest theologians I have consulted, until the work of Thomas Sanchez came to my hands."[37] The problem is, Moxius explains, that the seed cannot be expelled without titillation or some sense of pleasure, and "we" (speaking for the physicians) "anyhow expose ourselves to almost certain danger because of the friction of the genitals and the secretion of seed from these vessels—as happened to that widow according to Galen."[38] He therefore concludes that it is "illicit and indecorous" (*illicitum et indecorum*) for the physician to order such procedure to be executed: the spiritual harm outweighs any temporal gain.

The key issue for Moxius seems to be that as soon as the patient assents to the pleasure, she commits mortal sin; and even should she be strong enough to deny that assent, as Moxius puts it, out of love for Christ, "yet we expose ourselves to that danger and equally those whom we put in charge."[39] Galen's story of the widow proves to him that the mind is brought out of its senseless or unconscious state by the arousal by titillation, which affects both body and mind. He does not accept the casuistic distinction that the manipulation does not intend sexual pleasure or pollution and that these occur only *per accidens*, since excretion cannot be brought about without it.

I have condensed considerably Moxius's detailed and lengthy discussion, in which he takes up the more "liberal" Jesuit Sanchez' arguments point by point. Of all the physicians I have read on the subject of removing female seed, Moxius comes closest to acknowledging that the doctor-patient relationship might become questionable if the physician or his assistant in this manipulation gets aroused, and I have quoted the phrases that may suggest his awareness of that danger. All these passages, however, can be read as mere warnings not to become culpable by tempting the patient to sin. In the passage he takes from Sanchez (and which I cited) about unintended pollution occurring in the patient-surgeon encounter, it is not entirely clear, partly because of the scarcity of possessive pronouns in Latin, whose "pollution," or orgasm, is being imagined: the patient's or the surgeon's. Why was the physician's involvement as a potential threat to the physician-patient relationship not recognized or articulated more clearly? One reason might be that the female assistant, the *obstetrix*, imagined performing the manipulation in most of these situations was considered shield enough between female patient and physician (although the moral casuist Sanchez will in fact allow the physician to inspect the female body in exceptional cases),[40] but it could also be that not only was a vocabulary to express that change of doctor-patient relationship missing, but there was a sense of decorum making it close to impossible to talk about a physician's arousal, a sense of decorum, in fact, of which there are still remnants in our time. (One Renaissance way of obviating this decorum was, as we have seen, to speak not of a physician, but of a crude surgeon.)[41]

Unfortunately Moxius does not name the other "and without doubt most earnest theologians" who (as he claims) agree with him rather than with Sanchez. His words suggest that writers on moral-theological issues showed considerable interest in the treatment of the suffocation of the mother. It is noteworthy, however, that when he had been writing his *De Christiana ac tuta medendi ratione* (1591) two decades before Moxius's book, Battista Codronchi, as he was composing a major and detailed chapter on the ethics of the very treatment we are talking about, had specifically commented on the fact that he had been unable to find help from any *summista* for this difficult problem, suggesting that he found himself in novel territory as he was penning advice for his imagined "Christian physician." One would think that Codronchi would have looked for support quite carefully, since in the solution to this problem which he considered so difficult he found himself opposing "all the physicians" (*omnes Medici*)—thus Codronchi was unaware of Luis Mercado, whom I adduced above.[42]

Although, as I explained in my introduction, this subject lies outside the focus of my interest, it would seem that during the two decades that lie between the books of Codronchi and Moxius, the moral theologians took up the problem of how to cure this version of "hysteria." Finally it is also possible that because of Codronchi's distinct moral-theological bent, Moxius loosely included him among "the most earnest theologians" he had consulted, although, strictly speaking Codronchi was a physician.

Codronchi showed signs that he had truly wrestled with the ambiguity of the issue, even admitting that he once had felt differently about it: "Once I had thought that if the physician was quite sure that the hysteric was so senseless that she could not experience in that operation any kindling of pleasure or lust, and if it was a clear case of therapy and done for the good end and no scandal could arise from it, such defense could be tolerated."[43] He changed his mind when he realized that the physician could not be sure that the woman was entirely unconscious; therefore it was safer (*tutius*) to assume that she was conscious. And just as the physician could not for the sake of cure inebriate patients to have them empty their stomachs or join two deranged unmarried persons in sexual intercourse, he could not in this case have the female seed expelled without risking his eternal life. As we noticed before, there are indications that Rodrigo a Castro conceived his *Medicus-Politicus* at least in part as an answer or alternative to Codronchi's book on the Christian physician (although he does not refer to it), and it is therefore likely that Castro was familiar with Codronchi's opposition to this treatment of hysteria. If so, he may have put Codronchi, for whom he cannot have had much sympathy for a number of reasons (including his chapter against Jewish physicians), in one bag with the "wise men" he gently satirized.

But even if Castro may have had unexpressed reasons not to find Codronchi especially convincing, Codronchi's and Moxius's detailed argument against the procedure advocated in ancient medicine had a profound impact on Renaissance physicians even in Protestant countries. Daniel Sennert (1572–1637), the famous medical professor of Wittenberg, who influenced a large number of Protestant medical students in the seventeenth century, evidently accepted their objections, in spite of his respect for traditional medicine. Although he knows that Galen and Avicenna recommended titillation as a remedy, he judges that it is "doubtful" (very much a term of moral casuistry) whether that remedy can be prescribed and, after a

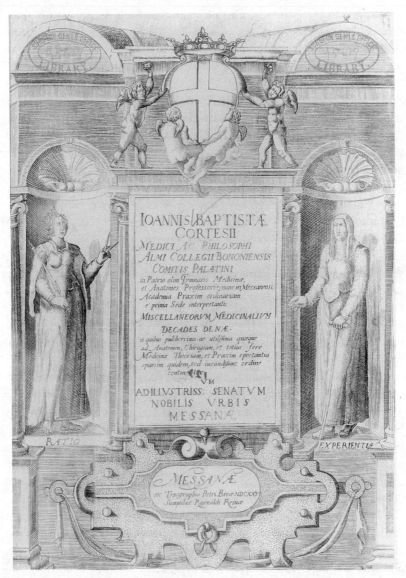

Figure 5.3. Frontispiece of Giovanni Battista Cortesi, *Miscellaneorum medicinalium decades*, Messanae, 1625 (National Library of Medicine).

discussion of the severity of various symptoms of the illness and finding that friction is applied instead of sexual activity (*Veneris vicem*), he judges: "It does not seem that it can be recommended by a Christian physician."[44] But rejection of the procedure was not universal: as

Audrey Eccles reports, Culpeper considered such scruples "foolish Popish superstition"; and while the English physician James Primrose made the bow (by this time almost standard) to the theologians, leaving them to decide "whether it is licit to help nature in this way in expelling semen," he cautiously but clearly indicated his sympathy with the *obstetrix* to help rid the patient of this "poison of the body" (*venenum corporis*): "It is not absurdly believed that it is allowed."[45]

Giovanni Battista Cortesi's response to Moxius is different in tone and substance from all the other discussions of *suffocatio ex retento semine*. Although Cortesi (1554–1636) does not challenge the traditional view of female seed, he assumes the air of the anatomist possessing firsthand knowledge of female genitalia, which he explains on several folio pages by means of detailed schematic cut-off illustrations. He lets his reader know that he gained his expertise in his youth by dissecting many bodies of young women.[46] Indeed in his unusual and distinguished career, Cortesi rose from humble barber and barber-surgeon to physician and professor of anatomy, first at Bologna, then (from 1599) at Messina.

"Before I touch on the matter itself," Cortesi says after quoting Moxius's view about what he considered the thorniest problem in contemporary medicine, "I need to prove that the solution of this problem does not pertain to the theologians whose counsel Moxius said he had sought, but is entirely the physicians' business, or rather something which theologians determine to be a matter of medicine."[47] The programmatic statement is followed by six folio pages explaining female physiology. Although he has earlier declared his preference for Hippocrates and Galen over Aristotle in the controversy concerning female seed, he sounds somewhat cautiously noncommittal at the end of this detailed exposition, when saying: "Whether that matter in the female testicles (*testes*) is semen or some residue (*excrementum*), as Aristotle said, is another matter."[48] He says correctly that all writers agree that semen should be ejected from the uterus, but that they disagree about the way this should be done: Sanchez proposes friction as a means and claims there is no need to worry if the woman is stirred to libido. "But it is one thing to consider the spoiled seed in the depth of the uterus, which can never be ejected through pleasure, and it is quite another to speak of the woman's seed contained in the spermatic vessels, particularly the testicles, from where it is indeed quite often emitted with pleasure."[49] The point of the distinction is that no amount of friction or titillation can flush the corrupted matter from the uterus, and a woman suffering from that condition will not experience relief from, or be healed by, an orgasm. In fact, Cortesi argues, not only can the traditionally advocated friction not bring about the emptying of the uterus of its spoilt matter, it can only add to it. The patient can only be given relief through the gentle finger of the midwife helping to empty the uterus—she may also use a pessary—and this without any danger of exciting the patient to pollution. Cortesi here backs up his suggestion by drawing on the down-to-earth Hippocrates for support, who said that sometimes not questions addressed to the patient but only the two fingers of the midwife could determine the state of the uterus. For a history of gynecology, it may be important to note that while Cortesi leaves the theory of female seed in place, he qualifies his language about the nature of the peccant fluid to allow for other possibilities. Thus he speaks of placing the pessary "where the spoiled seed is supposed to be" and of the origin of that fluid as "either originating within the space of the uterus or flowing from elsewhere through the open neck of the uterus."[50]

Cortesi very much doubts that the patient whom the moral casuist (and Jesuit) Sanchez is imagining, a woman between life and death, could experience pleasure if her clitoris were being handled. He takes a sharp shot at Moxius who, since he would not see or allow any other way of ridding the patient of the spoiled seed, advocated strong purgatives for her entire body: Cortesi surmises that in her condition they are more likely to kill her than help her. He calls the moral casuist Sanchez "inexperienced in anatomy" (*rei anatomiae haud peritus*, p. 818) if he thinks that the poisonous fluid can be evacuated by friction, for that is patently false. Then he adds: "But in my opinion more shameful still is the error of Moxius, who is a physician, when he assumes that in order to free the woman critically ill from her disease one must bring about a seminal flow."[51]

Thus Cortesi reclaims the matter for medicine, making the moral-theological question a medical one or substituting one for the other. But even in his terms, the controversy does not cease to be an ethical one. As the disagreement over the proper treatment is harnessed into the realm of medicine, it is placed on the scale of knowledge versus ignorance, and it follows that for a physician ignorance in medicine is shameful (*turpis*) or worse: by calling the physician's opinion and solution *turpius* (more shameful), he does not exculpate the opinion of the moral theologian venturing into the field of anatomy. By implication that foray remains shameful. Thus one may say that the problem of cure of this particular condition becomes one truly of *medical* ethics.

Removing the Male Seed

Diogenes, the Cynic philosopher, is known to have been the most self-controlled of all the people in regard to every act which required abstinence and endurance. However, he indulged in sexual relations, since he wanted to get rid of the inconvenience caused by the retention of sperm, but he did it not for pleasure associated with this elimination. Once he made an arrangement with a courtesan. But, as the story goes, when she came to him after some delay, he had already discharged the sperm by manual friction of his genitalia. After arrival he sent her away with the words: "My hand was faster than you in celebrating the bridal night." It is evident that a chaste person does not indulge in sexual intercourse for pleasure.[52]

This passage is from Galen and is immediately followed by Galen's account of curing the widow in the way we mentioned. Both passages are extremely well known in the Renaissance and are quoted and commented on by Zacuto.[53] It is almost universally believed in Renaissance Europe that the problem of relieving oneself of seed concerns both women and men, and Zacuto discusses both sides of the problem in one chapter. While the notion of seed may have an egalitarian effect (as modern historians have observed), there are, however, gender-specific differences: not only are the two types of seed different (the male variety hotter and stronger than the other), but there is a difference between the sexes (assumed to be as much physiological as resulting from habitual behavior) as to the need for venus. From the modern perspective the difference looks suspiciously like another version of the "double standard": while many males, particularly those leading a physically active life, inclining toward literature, and drinking with moderation, have the ability to convert seed to nutrition and therefore can do without sex without any danger to their health whatsoever, this is not so for women, as the sixteenth-century physician Duret tells us. "Since a woman lives in ease and has a body *dysdiaphoreton* ("hard to disperse," "not excreting readily"), she cannot live healthily if she does not have sex."[54] Duret backed up his view that for men sex is not essential for a healthy life with citations from Hippocrates.[55] The two main *loci classici*, however, for discussion of men's relief of seed are the Galenic passage about Diogenes quoted above and another from the end of *De locis affectis*, 6, about a friend of Galen's consulting him:

> A friend of mine who chose to completely refrain from intercourse contrary to his previous habits, developed such an inflated swelling of his penis that he felt the need to consult me about his symptoms. He said he was puzzled since athletes in perfect physical condition had a shriveled and collapsed penis, but he had the opposite condition, although he had abstained from sexual activity. I advised him to excrete the accumulated semen but afterward to refrain from [erotic] spectacles, not to tell stories or recall memories which could stimulate his sexual desire.
>
> In those persons who from early youth trained themselves in athletics and singing but remained entirely inexperienced in erotics and refrained from every thought and impression of it, the penis becomes small and shriveled as in old men. The same occurs in other people who as adolescents indulge for the first time in much venery. The blood vessels of their sexual organs become so dilated that their blood flows profusely in the vessels of these organs and increases ability and urge for intercourse.[56]

Abraham Zacuto, who continues to be my guide to what the Renaissance considers important, quotes both these Galenic passages in full in his chapter on the strangulation of the womb (or suffocation of the mother), proof enough, should any be needed, that the symptoms of female and male sexual abstinence were viewed together. Zacuto explains (somewhat tautologically) that the condition described in the case just quoted develops primarily in those who generate an abundance of seed and who, breaking with habit (*praeter consuetudinem*) abstain from coition, as well as in those who do not attempt to dissipate their seed by much exercise (vol. 1, p. 470). Expanding on Galen, he adds that athletes, farmers (*rurales*), and all others leading a hard-working life cure the excess of seed and blood by physical exercise.

Zacuto paraphrases Galen's story about Diogenes to point out that Diogenes used coition only at some intervals, and not for pleasure but for physical relief. He adds that he does not mean to deny that nature has linked pleasure with the act in order to secure the survival of the species, and that is why modest men (*modesti viri*) do not use intercourse merely for the sake of lust but for offspring. Possibly realizing that his moralizing has carried him far away from the anecdote about Diogenes, he now adds: "But why should Galen have called him most continent if, failing to wait for the prostitute, he satisfied himself relieving himself of sperm?"[57] For support for his moral censure, Zacuto then refers to Caelius Rhodiginus (Ludovico Ricchieri, 1450–1520) and to Roderigo a Castro, whom he here calls a "most famous physician" (*medicus celeberrimus*).

In Caelius Rhodiginus's well-known chapter on the practices of the Lydians, these are said to be acting as husbands without wife, a practice the Italian philologist and historian calls "shameful" (*turpis*).[58] Moral disapproval of such a practice (and also of Diogenes) is expressed even more strongly by Rodrigo a Castro. Commenting on Galen's anecdote about the Cynic, Castro had said that to some people Diogenes does not seem to have been a bad philosopher in that he used intercourse which "by the consensus of all good people" is to be used for offspring in order to avoid harm, but he was also "an extremely bad man" (*pessimus homo*).[59] While the humanistic notion of *consensus omnium bonorum* as the basis of a secular ethics is typical of the Castro I have described earlier, there is something elliptic and possibly deliberately obscure about this evaluation of Diogenes. It seems as if Castro would like to suggest that intercourse with the prostitute for release of seed is more excusable than masturbation (or rather that masturbation is less excusable)—although in the text of his treatise he does not quite bring himself to say so. But his own "scholion" to the passage expresses his extreme disgust for *masturbatores*.

The scholion is interesting for another matter: here Castro expresses not only his moral censure of masturbation, but also the medical writer's dilemma in being obliged to explain, though he may thereby mislead "lighter minds" (*leviores ingenii*). After noting that he knows no civil laws mentioning "this lasciviousness" (*istam lasciviam*), Castro lists or defines four kinds of what he calls "masturbation" and adds: "This I would have liked to have written only for the learned, and it is certainly to be omitted if someone should translate this book of [medical] praxis into the vernacular so that lighter and depraved minds are not shown the way to this most abject crime. And therefore I have compressed this scholion as much as I could, not so much for lack or barrenness of material but for the greatness of shame."[60] These are strong words of moral engagement not easily matched with the physician's feeling about other issues.

A Modern Misreading?

The topic of masturbation has received considerable attention in recent years. After commenting that "prohibitions against childhood masturbation are found in none of the primitive societies surveyed by Whiting and Child," says Lloyd DeMause in an essay often quoted: "The attitude of most people toward childhood masturbation prior to the eighteenth century can be seen in Fallopius's counsel for parents 'to be zealous in infancy to enlarge the penis of the boy.'"[61] This general view has been repeated and DeMause's opinion echoed by a number of scholars, particularly those interested in same-sex relationships in earlier periods. Thus Bruce R. Smith in his recent book on homosexuality in Shakespeare's time speaks of "the advice by Fallopius . . . and certain others that masturbation is healthy."[62] I submit that the quotation from Fallopius does not reveal anything about attitudes toward masturbation in the eighteenth nor in any other century, and I cannot find confirmation in medical works of the Renaissance that masturbation was considered healthy.

Of course there are Renaissance editors of Galen (for instance Tomás Rodriguez da Veiga, 1513–1579) who comment on almost everything except this aspect of Galen's recommendations—in view of Castro's difficulties in expressing himself, one would think out of some sense of decorum—although the tendency clearly is even for those most respectful of ancient medical authority to disagree. As that quotation from Castro has shown, masturbation is a matter not dealt with lightly. Sometimes there is an additional complication in the physicians' use of code words (like evacuation) that are euphemistic and ambiguous and certainly obscure the subject for the modern reader.

Thus Zacuto reprints and comments on a passage from Alzaharavius (or Albukasis), an Arabic physician of the tenth century, in which a paroxysm or fury is described that ceases when the patient emits semen. Alzahavarius adds that he encountered an adolescent suffering from that condition, whom he cured successfully. In his commentary on this passage, Zacuto refers to his own account of hysteria in women and adds that men similarly but more rarely show symptoms that cannot be mitigated except by excretion of seed (*non nisi excreto semine*).[63] He does not say how this is to be done. But a little later he speaks about how useful purgation (*purgatio*) is in such cases and surmises that an evacuation (*vacuatio*) was undoubtedly effected by Alzaharavius in this case. Apparently the matter of masturbation is so controversial that Zacuto prefers to remain ambiguous, for *vacuatio* could be a synonym for purgation or a code word for the excretion of semen, i.e., for masturbation (and is used in that sense by Rodriguez da Veiga in translating Galen).[64] In his important edition and commentary, Rodriguez da Veiga, incidentally, is long on physiological explanation but short on ethical evaluation of the ancient physician's recommendations.

As we have seen, retention of bad seed in women and men is viewed similarly except for the gravity and frequency of the condition. Although I have not found a passage in Moxius that directly addresses the use of male masturbation for curing, I would very much doubt that Moxius, so opposed to the use of *fricatio* of female pudenda, even in situations he considered life threatening, would allow it in men. A somewhat indirect passage taken from the context of cure of female hysteria confirms my view. After speaking of retained seed, Moxius moves to corrupted seed thus:

> But he [Galen] thinks those conditions more lethal which are caused by the corrupt seed in the same way in members of both sexes. For the following epigram by Angelo Poliziano about Michael Morino shows that this happens also in men:
> Sola Venus poterat lento succurrere morbo:
> Ne se poluerit, maluit ille mori.
> (Only Venus could relieve his slow disease.
> In order not to pollute himself, he rather died.)[65]

For the Renaissance audience, the epigram would have gained in significance through the widely circulating rumor that the brilliant humanist and poet Angelo Poliziano (1454–1494) had killed himself, distraught about his love for a young man. Whether Poliziano's rumored death was actually a suicide or not, the epigram itself as quoted by Moxius presents death as preferable to any sexual relief considered illicit, including masturbation. Thus it can hardly be said that Moxius advocates masturbation.

I have not detected a difference of emphasis between Protestant and Catholic physicians with respect to masturbation. Obviously the

Jewish physician Rodrigo a Castro, trained in Spain and writing in Protestant Hamburg, condemns it. The eminent Protestant physician Daniel Sennert, professor at Wittenberg, whose book *Epitome institutionum medicinae* was eventually even translated into English, writes in a chapter entitled "De Excretis, et Retentis, ac Venere":

> Unseasonably retained seed brings about slowness and sluggishness of the body, and if the seed deteriorates, it causes the most serious symptoms, which it is proper to avoid by sexual activity. But this should be proper and lawful. For there is no need to try something for the preservation of health that is contrary to divine laws; and the Creator has provided man with as much in this matter as is necessary to avoid all that is detrimental to health.[66]

Sennert's sensibility, like Rodrigo a Castro's, has undoubtedly been formed by the Old Testament and its condemnation of masturbation. (At least thus was the story of Onan [Gen. 38], perhaps more properly a case of *coitus interruptus*, interpreted.) If we remember that for Melanchthon the Old Testament with its divine laws was in fact synonymous with the laws of nature, we may understand that Sennert was most likely not aware of making a statement on Christian ethics but was thinking in terms of general ethics, i.e. writing in the role he thought proper for a physician; in other words, he was talking of the natural laws by which all sciences were bound.

With the sociologist Norbert Elias as its most prominent proponent, there is currently a view of the general course of civilization as a process of restricting earlier or "primitive" freedom, particularly with respect to shame and nudity, and one may wonder how early modern proscriptions of masturbation fit into such a general scheme. DeMause's observation about how earlier ages condoned it in children (with which I opened this section) could be aligned with it perfectly. It is exactly against such a view of civilization, however, that Hans Peter Duerr recently published two impressive tomes on many subjects that relate to my study.[67] Duerr proves convincingly, if it needed proof, that earlier civilizations were more restrictive than our own in important aspects relating to sex and nudity (for instance childbirth, bathing habits, and taboos about defecation). But while Duerr makes some extremely interesting observations about practices of baring and displaying a child's penis in various periods and cultures (and finds, incidentally, that there are no comparable practices of baring a young girl's genitalia), he does not address the topic of masturbation. Thus we are on our own in determining how Fallopius and other Renaissance physicians viewed this matter.

The sentence quoted by DeMause is from Fallopius's work *De decoratione*. The title invokes associations with *decorum*, in the Renaissance sometimes translated as "seemliness" or as "proportion." But rather than being about decorum in the sense of seemly behavior of the physician, it is about the seemliness and proportion of the human body and about how the physician can contribute (by prescribing corrective diet, exercise, etc.) to bringing about its most pleasing shape and function. Disproportion may be the result of nature (birth), illness, or accident.

In chapter 17 (from which DeMause's quotation is taken), as in the rest of the book, the perspective Fallopius adopts is not merely aesthetic (focusing on beauty and the harmony of body parts) or epicurean (achieving the greatest pleasure), but clearly medical-teleological: How can the body parts designed for procreation best fulfill their purpose? Thus Fallopius says that he feels it is his duty to write about the size of the male member of generation, the penis, a subject he says modern physicians do not treat since humanity has now turned more bashful (*honestius*) and does not look at the body nude anymore—in antiquity all parts of the body were often seen both in the gymnasium and in the bath. And if some severe and dour people (*taetrici viri*) should object to his treating ways of enlarging the penis, since they think the matter shameful (*turpis*) for a physician, he would reply that everything he is doing is to help preserve the species. For if the male member is not enclosed properly by the vulva, the woman does not experience pleasure and does not emit semen, hence conception does not happen. It is at this point that he says: "I encourage parents to attempt to enlarge the member of their boys in childhood" (*aetas infantilis*).[68] A little further down, and after referring to Avicenna for support, he says how this should be done: using various ointments, one should rub the child's penis. The hints he gives for facilitating the procedure may help us imagine the scene and determine whether the action can be called masturbation, in any sense:

For these reasons, rubbing transversely, we extend the member. This is also done with warming utensils like hot water bottles placed between the legs or warm towels. But make sure that as soon as the penis becomes feeble, you bring it to erection again by warm towels or something else warm; for that helps the boys and even the other people present [or: and even older ones, *et etiam consistentibus*]. But one should take care with the weak ones, who do not have an abundance of spirit, lest they not be able to fill the swollen vessels with spirit. That should be remedied by medications suggested by practical physicians.[69]

This is the context of Fallopius's suggestion to the parents. (To understand the physiology informing the passage, we must recall that according to traditional theory, three elements were necessary for sexual performance: semen, heat, and pneuma, here called "spiritus.") We notice that before the medical author gets to his subject, he indicates his awareness that he is treading on dangerous ground: he is defensive as he justifies a subject considered shameful (we might say "tabooed"). The context of the suggested manipulation has been translated in detail to give an impression of what scene we need to imagine: children of *aetas infantilis*, i.e. small children, surrounded by those Fallopius calls *consistentes*, a word that (according to DuCange's dictionary of medieval Latin) meant people present or praying at a ceremony. They would have included parents, nurses, and perhaps other helpers. But I admit that I am less sure of this translation than I should be and therefore, in the quotation above, suggest an alternative reading. The meaning of *panna* is "swaddling clothes," but also any pieces of cloth, like towels, which in this case would be warmed, and I was tempted to translate it with the anachronistic word "diapers" to suggest the nature of the scene. In any case, whatever interpretation one adopts, neither the manipulation itself nor its medical justification have much if anything to do with masturbation.

In his most interesting chapter entitled "The Sexuality of Children," a brief survey of attitudes of different periods and cultures, the sociologist Hans Peter Duerr points to the right context of such practices when saying, "The future monarch's capacity for erection is a matter of state interest."[70] Fallopius's intent is apparently not only to develop the member's size but to detect weakness early in order to remedy it by drugs. After describing the manipulation, Fallopius puts the matter in perspective a second time in a similar manner: "What I am saying and yet am going to say I am constrained to speak in the interest of childbearing—not that I would dare to advocate anything against the law or against good morals."[71] At the same time a sentence as defensive as this is an index, as I said, that Fallopius knows he is moving in dangerous territory, namely that the advocated practice might be interpreted as violating accepted morals. Fallopius's sentence thus does not show that accepted morals did not cover children's masturbation (or that he even encouraged it), but quite the contrary.

The modern historian may have difficulty grasping the specifics of a medical theory that made Fallopius advocate practices which, transferred into the different paradigm of twentieth-century medicine, may seem grotesque. Yet the theory (which I summarized above) is there for anyone curious enough to find out. Fallopius makes the point that his overriding concern is corrective, and this is also true as he advocates gentle massaging of women's breasts that are underdeveloped.[72] That this physician who lectured about the details of *pudenda* or *verenda* with more candor and precision than most professors of his day occasionally butted against taboos, and that for him medical reasoning in some manner was bounded by theological reasoning, can be seen from a passage in which he wonders why God required His people to cut their foreskin: "But if someone asks why the Most High God in his elected people instituted the cutting of the prepuce, the reasons are eternal and rest in the mind of the Most High and are not to be discussed in secular schools."[73] Perhaps in lectures Fallopius left the matter at this rhetorical figure of omission (*praeter-itio*); in the work as printed in 1600, probably a lecture transcript, he continues, after a square bracket inserted by the printer, with some speculations that may or may not be the ones unsuitable for "secular schools": possibly God ordered the cutting because the prepuce increases sexual pleasure, from which God wanted his people to abstain as much as possible (so that they would not neglect worshiping him). Fallopius speculates that the foreskin may be the reason why Jewish, Turkish, and Mauritanian women are said to sleep with Christian slaves rather than with their circumcised lords. But he adds that those who have the gland bared are more rarely infected by syphilis (*lues gallica*).[74]

In his recommendations for strengthening the male organ as in those for expanding women's breasts, Fallopius' declared aim is not or not merely some standard of beauty, but proper functioning in producing and sustaining offspring (*non tantum ratione pulchritudinis,*

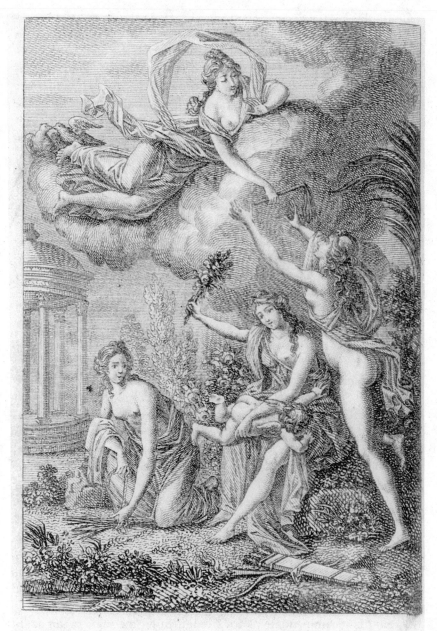

Delicias parunt Veneri crudelia flagra,
Dum nocet, illa juvat, dum juvat ecce nocet.

Figure 5.4.   Johann Heinrich Meibom, *A Treatise on the Use of Flogging in Venereal Affairs*, London, 1718 (with permission of the Folger Shakespeare Library).

J. H. MEIBOMII,

DE

FLAGRORUM USU

IN RE MEDICA ET VENEREA,

ET LUMBORUM RENUMQUE OFFICIO.

EDENTE

CLAUDIO MERCIER, COMPENDIENSI.

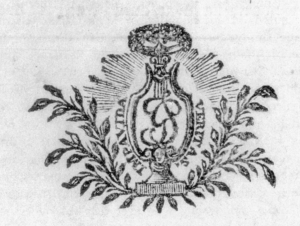

PARISIIS,

SUMPTIBUS JAC. GIROUARD.

M. DCC. XCII.

Figure 5.4   continued

quantum ratione foetus),[75] understandably, of course, since having off-spring was the prime purpose of marriage. We saw that the recommendation about how to strengthen a male child's member is addressed to parents and that the advocated manipulation, different from anything one would call "masturbation," is to be done in the context of the family. It would seem that we are here catching a glimpse of the post-Reformational emphasis on the family that cultural historians have observed on all sides of the religious spectrum. But there can be no doubt that the effects of that development were felt first and foremost in Protestant countries, to which I intend to return once more to study how even sexual practices at the margin of what was known or imaginable could be harnessed into the marital bond.

On the Margin of Sexual Stimulation: Meibom

In 1639, Johann Heinrich Meibom (Meibomius), whom I have cited before as author of one of the most learned commentaries on the Hippocratic oath, wrote a letter, "On the Use of Flogging in Medical and Venereal Affairs: The Functions of the Reins and Loins." This Latin *epistola*, first published in 1639 at Leyden, was often reprinted and eventually translated into German and English. Medical letters partake, of course, of the epistolary or "low" style, they are not treatises, and the physician Meibom in his first sentence reminds his addressee, a bishop at Lübeck and privy councillor to the Duke of Holstein, that he has promised him this piece of writing "over a bottle." Yet there is a long tradition of medical letter writing (true or faked—such as the pseudo-Hippocratic letters), necessarily composed as *sermo* and dealing with everyday occurrences and cases. Meibom's letter belongs to this very respectable genre, and is of inestimable value for anyone interested in the medical ethics of a previous period. It strikes me therefore that the letter as originally printed has a different place, context, and therefore meaning from the version "made English from the Latin original by a Physician," which I will use for my quotations.[76] This English version of 1718 is prefaced by an engraving of a male on his knees; he is being flogged on his bare behind by a young female servant while another woman is waiting expectantly on a bed. (The Folger Library copy is bound with other works of 1718 from the same notorious London printer E. Curll, including the anonymous *Treatise of Hermaphrodites* attributed to Giles Jacob.) This edition more clearly belongs to the genre sometimes called "curious" and including the pornographic, which used to require special classification.[77] Meibom's Latin *epistola*, however, is not primarily pornography, though it is informal and meant to be enjoyable for its addressee; with its detailed physiological reasoning, it is informed by the medical and, as I will argue, ultimately also ethical interests of its author.

Meibom first surveys traditional medical uses of flogging, as in the treatment of melancholics and madmen, but soon zeroes in on the topic of beating as sexual stimulus. He reports the view (of Monytius Taventius) "that if Sterility is suspected from the shortness of the *Penis* that the Defect may be amended, and the Part extended by the Use of that Discipline" (p. 6), and remembers that Petronius has the same prescription for curing languid ineptness. He then cites in varying detail five cases of men who depended on flogging for performance in coition. They derive from Giovanni Pico della Mirandola; Caelius Rhodiginus (Ludovico Ricchieri) through André Tiraqueau; Otto Brunfels' *Onomastikon sive lexikon medicinae* (1st ed., 1534); from his own informants in the city of Lübeck, in which he lived for thirty years and was "Stadtphysikus" ("a new and late instance," p. 11); and his reading about Holland (a case "not many years since," which I will omit, since it adds little to the others).

Here is the first example in the somewhat distracting language of the eighteenth-century translation:

> Johannes Picus . . . in his 3d Book *against the Astrologers*, Chap. 27 relates this of an Acquaintance of his, "There is now alive, says he, a Man of a prodigious, and almost unheard kind of Lechery: For he is never inflamed to Pleasure, but when he is wipt; and yet he is so intent on the Act, and longs for the Strokes with such an Earnestness, that he blames the Flogger that uses him gently, and is never thoroughly Master of his Wishes unless the Blood starts, and the Whip rages smartly o'er the wicked Limbs of the Monster. This Creature begs this Favour of the Woman whom he is to enjoy, brings her a Rod himself, soak'd and harden'd in Vinegar a Day before for the same Purpose, and intreats the Blessing of a Whipping from the Harlot [*meretrix*] on his Knees; and the more smartly he is whipt, he rages the more eagerly, and goes the same Pace both to Pleasure and Pain. A singular Instance of one who finds Delight in the midst of Torment; and as he is not a Man very vicious in other Respects, he acknowledges his Distemper, and abhors it." (pp. 7–9)

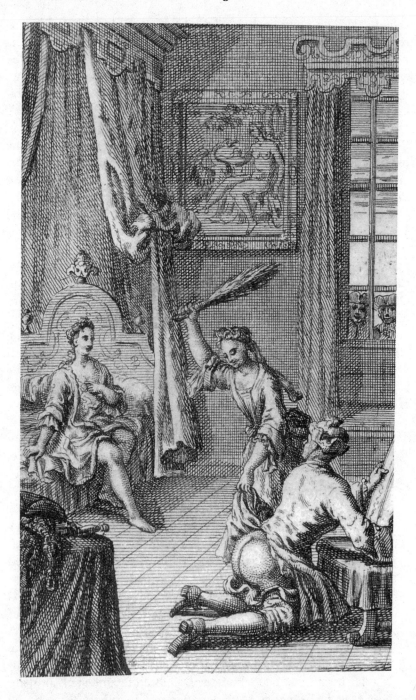

Figure 5.5.   Illustration of Johann Heinrich Meibom, *De flagrorum usu in re medica et venerea*, Paris, 1792 (National Library of Medicine).

A

TREATISE

Of the USE of

FLOGGING

In Venereal Affairs:

ALSO

Of the OFFICE of the

LOINS and REINS.

Written to the Famous CHRISTIANUS
CASSIUS, Bishop of *Lubeck*, and Privy-
Councellor to the Duke of *Holstein*.

By JOHN HENRY MEIBOMIUS, M.D.

Made *English* from the *Latin* Original
By a PHYSICIAN.

Delicias pariunt Veneri *crudelia* Flagra;
Dum nocet, illa juvat; dum juvat, ecce nocet.

To which is Added,
A TREATISE of HERMAPHRODITES.

LONDON,
Printed for E. CURLL, in *Fleet-street*, 1718. Price 3*s.*
Where may be had,
The CASES of IMPOTENCY, and EUNUCHISM
and ONANISM Display'd, in 7 Vols. Price 18*s.*

Figure 5.5   continued

While this is clearly an account of an extramarital relationship, Meibom's second case (from Caelius Rhodiginus) is ambiguous in that respect:

> It is certain upon the Oath of credible Persons, that not many years since there lived a Man not of a Salaciousness, resembling Cocks, but of a more wonderful, and almost incredible sort of Lechery; who the more Stripes he received, was the more violently hurried to Coition. The Case was prodigious, since it was a Question which he desired most, the Blows or the Act itself, unless the Pleasure of the last was measured by the Number of the former: Besides it was his Manner to heighten the Smartness of the Rod with Vinegar the Day before it was to be used, and then to request the Discipline with violent Entreaties. But if the *Flogger* seemed to work slowly, he flew into a Passion, and abused him. He was never contented unless the Blood sprung out, and followed the Lash; a rare Instance of a Man who went with an equal pace to Pleasure and to Pain and who, in the midst of Torture, either satisfied or excited a pleasing Titulation (sic), and a furious itch of Lust. (p. 9–10)

The third case, according to Meibom from Otto Brunsfels' medical dictionary (under the word "coition"), is about a married man at Munich "who never could enjoy his Wife, if he was not soundly flogged to it before he made his Attempts" (p. 11). To these cases Meibom adds a "late instance" from his home city about a married man's relationship with a prostitute:

> A Citizen of *Lübeck*, a Cheesemonger by Trade, living in the *Millers*-Street was cited before the Magistrates, among other Crimes, for Adultery; and the Fact being proved, he was banished. A Courtesan with whom this Fellow had often an Affair, confessed before the Deputies of the Senate, that he could never have a forcible Erection, and perform the Duty of a Man, 'till she had whipped him on the Back with Rods; and that when the Business was over, that he could not be brought to a Repetition, unless excited by a second Flogging. (p. 11)

Meibom next inquires into the causes of such proclivities and (after rejecting, with Pico, the influence of the stars) also highlights Pico's explanation that the subject of that case (according to his own word) was educated "with a Number of wicked Boys [*pueri scelestissimi*], who set up this Trade of Whipping among themselves, and purchased each other these infamous Stripes at the Expense of Modesty" (p. 14). Meibom points out that Caelius Rhodiginus has a similar explanation, which he goes on to quote:

> Nor is it less wonderful, that this uncommon Vice should be known by the Person; and that he should hate and condemn himself for it; but by the Force of a vicious Habit gaining ground upon him, he practic'd a Vice he disapprov'd. But it grew more obstinate and rooted in Nature, from his using it from a Child (*puer*), when a reciprocal Frication among his School-Fellows (*inter aequales*) used to be provoked by the Titulaton of Stripes. A strange Instance what a Power the Force of Education has in grafting inveterate ill Habits on our Morals. (pp. 14–15)

The modern reader may find aspects of this explanatory attempt quite perceptive, and I for one remember that at one of those all-male schools in Meibom's home town three and a half centuries after him, some of my classmates on the way to or from the shower would sometimes (in a jest that was not necessarily interpreted as sexual) try to smack a towel on each other's behind or genitals. But Meibom has a different explanation in mind. "So far they," he says—i.e. that is what they can offer toward explanation; he is willing to give their idea some credence and takes into account that Aristotle in his *Ethics* thinks of custom as "a sort of second nature" (p. 15). He further concedes that in the instances of Pico and Caelius Rhodiginus custom "might contribute something to the Cause" (p. 15). But the cases from Brunfels (about the Munich husband) and the one from his own experience in Lübeck do not fit this explanation: although he does not say so, they presumably are different because those men did not grow up in what the English translator calls "a youthful Fraternity" (p. 16), i.e. as *pueri eiusdem sodalitatis* (1643 ed., p. 16) of some academy. Even more important, why did the others of that "youthful fraternity" not develop the same tastes as Pico's acquaintance? Custom, it seems, has only a selective effect: "Neither is it probable that all those Boys we mentioned began their Youth with exposing their Chastity to sale, with this reciprocal Communication of Vice, and used Rods at the first to provoke Lechery" (p. 16). The passage that follows may be taken as a mere self-congratulatory piece of homophobia, but it is interesting in my context, revealing not only how this physician in the early seventeenth century viewed male same-sex relationships, but also masturbation.[78] Particularly singling out the sexual activities of boys, he says: "I congratulate our *Germany*, that these Vices of perverse Lust, these Disgraces of Children (*pueri*) and mutual Pollutions of Males, are almost unknown amongst us, and if by accident such Case happens, the Offenders are severely punished, by being burnt for their Crimes" (p. 16). Having established to his satisfaction that "neither the Stars nor Custom are the Cause why Stripes excite Venery," he thus feels urged (in a clever rhetorical move) to look for an explanation elsewhere.

His solution, in itself of little interest in my context, lies in his perceiving a close connection of the kidneys (our translator says "reins") and the whole area of the lower back ("loins") with the genitalia through nerves, arteries, and "seminal veins." He argues this point both with the help of historical philology (showing how words for reins and loins in Greek literature and in the Bible are used to signify the place of generation—a weak argument since he seems to disregard euphemistic use of language) and with classical and contemporary medicine. As to the medical-physiological argument (its elaborateness confirms my view that this epistle was not mere tongue-in-cheek pornography), he points to an anatomist who found as he dissected a man known for his sexual exploits that he had kidneys "of a prodigious size." More than on anyone else, he relies on Sennert in emphasizing the connection between kidneys and semen: that a kidney disorder can result from retention of seed, that signs of warm kidneys indicate sexual drive, and that practitioners can deduce the quality of the semen from the constitution of the kidneys. Thus he finally concludes "that Strokes upon the *Back* and *Loins* as Parts appropriated for the Generating of Seed, and carrying it to the Genitals, warm and inflame those Parts, and contribute very much to the Irritation of *Lechery*" (p. 50). Pointing out this nexus was no doubt what Meibomius considered his primary contribution.

But the Lübeck physician does not leave matters at that. Possibly he sees his contribution as restricted not to what we might now call psychopathology but as having broader significance or application; or it is his profound interest in medical ethics (a few years later, he was to publish one of the most learned commentaries on the Hippocratic oath ever written)[79] that makes him continue:

This, dear *Cassius*, is my Opinion; but you will object that the Persons I treat of, are such as being exhausted by a licentious Venery, made Use of this Remedy, for the Continuation of their ungovernable Lusts, and a Repetition of the same filthy Enjoyments. But then you ask, since the Case is so, whether a Person, who has practis'd *Lawful Love*, and yet perceives his *Loins* and *Sides* languid (the Subject of this Treatise) may not without the Imputation of any Crime, make use of the same Method, in order to discharge a Debt which I won't say is due, but to please the Creator? (p. 51–52)

His answer is an unqualified "yes." He is certain that his addressee (whose wife is pregnant at the time of his writing) will not need such stimuli: "However, I won't forbid[80] you communicating this Remedy to others who may have Occasion for a *Flogger*." Of all "professors of science," he says with a Greek proverb, physicians are expected to be particularly open and broad-minded; and he ends with a sentence from Scribonius Largus (first century A.D.) addressed to Julius Calistus, that chastises envy[81] and instead holds up pity and humaneness as the prime criteria by which to judge all people, but most especially physicians.

The issues reviewed in this chapter are on the margin of what was expressible by Renaissance physicians. For that very reason they are interesting to us. To the achievements of Renaissance sexology (the precision of the description of the female organs by Fallopius, Cortesi, and others, together with the rejection by the "neoterici" of Galen's notion of inside-out correspondence and comparison of male and female genitalia), earlier in this chapter I added another: a growing sensitivity to the moral issues raised for those involved in manipulating female genitalia (going beyond the traditional notions of modesty and shame). My claim may have seemed bold, overblown, or partial, and my addition incongruous with the other achievements mentioned. Some clarification may be in order.

Terms like sensitivity are potentially loaded and reversible. More objectively put, physicians of the later Renaissance comment more extensively on the ethics of their intervention than do their predecessors (for instance, Grado and Guainerio). I may have shown insensitivity to the plight of women at the mercy of the (male) physician, and it may be argued (I do not know how cogently) that the problems discussed with increased sensitivity are ultimately male problems, not women's issues. Perhaps female patients in the Middle Ages were better off than those in the Renaissance if, as Monica Green has suggested in an important review essay, more of them received their health care from women, no matter whether called midwives, *obstetrices*, matrons, *mulierculae*, or *sages femmes*, whose role was not restricted to midwifing.[82] For from another perspective the issues reviewed in the first half of this chapter represent the struggles of academically trained physicians to master areas of gynecology in which they had not necessarily claimed expertise before. The word "master" suggests a power struggle, naively the battle of the sexes, more concretely the physicians' attempts to oust the *mulierculae*.[83] But *master* also means control by knowledge, understanding, research; and as limited as Renaissance medicine may have been, the history of modern gynecology is in some way continuous with it: knowledge may have progressed by leaps and bounds, but modern gynecology derives from Renaissance versions of it. The treatment of one variety of what in that period was called "hysteria," namely the one thought to be caused by spoilt seed, shows how academic physicians dealt with an area of the female body they were still forbidden to touch. The *obstetrix*, in an agreement that is surprisingly general, serves as the intermediary to perform the manipulation. Since, except for some lecture transcripts, the works used are carefully crafted for print, it would be hasty to draw conclusions about actual practice, but it cannot be an accident that the two cases in which the operating taboo is violated and the privacy of the female body invaded by a male, the perpetrator is a surgeon serving as a negative example of how not to proceed. It should also be noted that in one of the cited examples the crude surgeon is executing a version of an invasive and violent practice that Foreest assigns to ignorant and shameless *mulierculae*.

Given the traditional legitimation of sexual activity through the act of generation and given also the importance of volition or consent to an act defined as sin, it should not be surprising that Renaissance speculation about the legitimacy of the manipulation advocated by ancient medicine focuses on the patient's level of consciousness and her ability to experience pleasure. If that focus seems arcane to modern readers, that impression may be an index of how far they are removed from older ways of Christian thinking. Although the precedent of non-Christian medical authorities advocating the usefulness of the procedure is powerful (Sennert mentions Galen and Avicenna), Roman Catholic physicians like Mercato, Codronchi, Moxius, and

Ranchin rejected the manipulation on the grounds of moral theology, and it is no doubt because of their rejection and argumentation also that the Protestant Sennert not only rejects it but calls that rejection proper to the "Christian physician." It is tempting to see this new ethical sense, antagonistic to traditional authorities (Galen and Avicenna), as part of the general undermining of Galen's and Avicenna's physiology that Owsei Temkin and Nancy Siraisi have described for the period. But the fact that Mercato, Codronchi, Moxius, Ranchin, and even the Protestant Sennert are Galenists (although Sennert made an attempt to harmonize or update Galenism with chemical, i.e. Paracelsian, medicine) gives me pause. More likely the explanation lies in an upsurge of ethical interest in the wake of the Reformation and Counter-Reformation, and the first impulse would thus be outside the parameters of this study.[84] The tide had clearly turned against the "liberal" moral casuist Sanchez, who (in the paragraph that ignited Moxius' disagreement) claimed to have checked the matter with the most learned of the Jesuits. While Sanchez' large work on conjugal ethics went through many editions with hardly any changes, the entire paragraph discussing the ethical appropriateness of the therapy in question (tom. 3, lib. 9, disput. 17, num. 19) was dropped in the Antwerp edition (1614) after his death and from the subsequent (Antwerp) editions deriving from it.[85] The revision, obscured by a careful renumbering of paragraphs, may signify a recognition that Sanchez's opinion on a controverted topic was considered out of line with "Christian physicians" or else it may be proof that Cortesi's physiological critique had been taken to heart.

In most of these discussions, distinctions are made between different kinds of women to whom the procedure is to be applied or not applied. Galen singled out widows, and widows keep being the primary target group, together with *moniales* (nuns), from Grado through Foreest (in Holland) to Rodrigo a Castro (in Protestant Hamburg), an index that we are to some extent dealing with medical commonplaces. With Foreest, among other physicians, we saw a tendency to exclude young women: married ones for reasons we noted in Foreest and *nubiles* (since it is assumed that they could or should get married). Together with some obvious gender paradigms, medical reasons (possibly about the orgasm to be stimulated) in such discussions begin to be combined with ethical ones that still need to be emphasized because they are easily overlooked. In her instructive essay on Antonio Guainerio's *Tractatus de matricibus*, Helen Lemay summarizes the cure for the suffocation of the uterus from Guainerio, a version of the digital titillation (by a midwife) we have been describing, and adds: "He comments that the midwife will be more successful in this procedure if the patient is not a virgin, although it is not necessary if she is married. . . ."[86] The Latin passage, which I give in the notes, seems to suggest that with a *mulier corrupta* the midwife will be more successful in inserting her finger into "the neck of the womb" (*matricis collum*).[87]

It would seem that with Guainerio (who is very early in my context—he died about 1448) this is a medical comment about the relative ease of producing an orgasm to eject the noxious fluids; it is not—or at least not primarily—a statement informed by the ethical sense that virginity requires restraint. Later in the period, physicians will feel that this stimulation to orgasm is a violation of virginity and therefore oppose it. Francois Ranchin, so often at the cutting edge of feelings about medical ethics, will write in a section entitled, "Whether One Is Allowed to Rub the Vulva of Women in Hysterical Paroxysm?": "We, however, following the theologians, hold such friction to be abominable and damnable, particularly in virgins, since such pollution may spoil virginity."[88] After these strong words, Ranchin adds that, although women other than virgins may present different cases, he still would not recommend the procedure to "Christian physicians." It may even be that the conditional clause used by Rodrigo a Castro in this context, which I highlighted earlier ("if that can be done without crime") is not quite as ethically imprecise (and perhaps "hedging") as I took it to be, but refers to these distinctions: it would be a crime (*scelus*) to do this to a virgin.

If I have not been able to limit myself entirely to medical authors, it is partly because moral-theological writers occasionally figure in medical discourse. But they are not allowed to blend in homogeneously, as we saw in Cortesi's discussion, who is very much aware of who is a physician and who is not (and awards blame for ignorance of physiology accordingly). By unhooking the traditional nexus between physiological cause and psychological consequence, this gynecological expert, who gained his expertise by dissecting bodies of women, claims the gynecological area for the physician, thus removing the theologian. It is true that his bold move leaves intact the boundaries or margins of modesty that we observed: for even Cortesi is careful to point out that the different operation he advocates (which did not involve titillation) is executed by a woman *obstetrix*.

But the medicalization and concomitant secularization of the treatment is nevertheless significant.

Given the high regard so-called rational physicians had for Galen in the Renaissance, their strong disagreement with his admiration for Diogenes, or more specifically, their disagreement with his evaluation of Diogenes' way of finding sexual relief, is surprising. While their critique of Galen's way of ridding female patients of spoiled seed is sometimes articulate, it is not general and arises late in the period; as for males, i.e. for male seed, the Renaissance physicians' disagreement with Galen is general: any medical writer who touches at all on the subject of masturbation seems to condemn it. While (because of the common etiology) the problem of ridding the patient of spoiled seed is essentially conceived as the same for males and females, there are important differences relating to the Renaissance conception of gender, which I need not repeat here. It should be noted, though, that what we previously observed to be margins of shame or modesty enveloping the female body appear in treatments of this topic as margins of expression or expressibility: what are physiological margins of shame with one topic are linguistic margins of shame with the other. As they enter into the topic or leave it, Renaissance medical authors suggest not only that they are extremely uncomfortable with the subject, but that they cannot or should not express it. We saw Rodrigo a Castro's "solution" of the problem of inexpressibility in his attempt, real or pretended, to create two audiences: a general audience, learned enough to read his Latin treatise, and the specialized readers to whom, in addition, his scholia are addressed. His concern to keep his scholion from being translated may be real, although his attempt to divide his Latin-speaking readership, i.e. his attempt to construct two audiences, must remain merely theoretical. But whether the concern about wrong addressees is genuine or pretended, practical or theoretical, its expression allows Castro to speak about what is strongly tabooed, since it overlaps (as his division into kinds of masturbation indicates) with "that matter which ought not to be heard of" in the period, homosexual acts.[89]

It is undoubtedly because of this nexus that DeMause's statement about older views on children's masturbation has received considerable attention, although that statement is based on a single sentence from a Renaissance physician. In my view that sentence has been misread by being taken out of its original context, which is not masturbation. As we saw, Fallopius, entering into his topic and leaving it, tries to make it clear that he is not talking about masturbation, stimulation of the sexual organ by oneself. For what could be the shameful activity with which he would not want the recommended one confused other than some form of masturbation? In any case Fallopius's sentence is a weak prop for generalizing statements about Renaissance attitudes. Sexual stimulations of young boys also has a place in Meibom's report of others' attempts at explaining how some persons became attracted to what we now call masochistic behavior as sexual stimulant: of course Meibom also views the sexual stimulation of boys as highly negative. Thus, if I were to generalize on the basis of limited data, my opinion would be the opposite of DeMause's: the Renaissance (to judge from what physicians write) is extraordinarily uneasy about masturbation, including children's masturbation, and that unease may be fed by perceived links with homosexual acts. In this respect Meibom, whatever the level of seriousness of his epistle, is far from unusual: his comments on the history of same-sex relationships here and elsewhere agree perfectly with the homophobic strain that can be perceived in Renaissance Europe in general and Protestant countries in particular. If Protestantism emphasized the value of marriage and (as C. S. Lewis has shown so memorably) romance was from now on only imaginable as leading to marriage, homophobia in some sense is the other side of this coin.

What is unusual about Meibom is the ethical question he raises at the end of his letter about flogging and the answer he proposes and justifies. My point is that Meibom's homophobic history of sexuality has a "deep" link with his originality. In the realm of sexual practices on the margin of what was imaginable for most of his contemporaries, Meibom (son of a minister) in a letter to his friend (a Lutheran churchman) makes physicians the epitome of understanding. He integrates these marginal practices into conjugal relations. As he does, it would seem that he is outdoing the man of the cloth, whose objections he conceives at least as possible, by not using terms heavily fraught with Christian resonance (like *caritas*), but by requiring classical ethical qualities which may predate Christian virtues and from which the notion of *Christus:medicus* may in effect be said to derive its power (see Mt. 9:13, among other passages): he urges that (in terms appropriated from a non-Christian physician) the physician's mind (*animus*) more than anyone else's, *plenus sit mesericordiae et humanitatis* (be filled with pity and humaneness). It would thus appear that Meibom of Lübeck writes in the secular tradition of medical ethics strongly professed by Rodrigo a Castro of Hamburg.

NOTES

1. *Sexuality and Medicine in the Middle Ages,* trans. Matthew Adamson (Princeton, N. J.: Princeton University Press, 1985), p. 61.

2. Hippocrates, *De generatione,* 4 (ed. Littré [Paris: Baillière, 1851], vol. 7, p. 475). Quoted from Jacquart and Thomasset, *Sexuality and Medicine,* p. 62.

3. Valesius, *Controversiarum medicarum et philosophicarum,* 3d ed. (Frankfurt, 1590), lib. 2, chap. 7 (p. 71): "Sed dicet aliquis: (nam quae a vulgaribus philosophis hinc inde dicuntur contemno) Si utrumque semen, utrumque praestaret; posset foemina sine concubitu, ex seipsa concipere. Quo nil videtur absurdius. Respondendum, Muliebre semen, etiam si res habeat, ut diximus, tamen minoris esse virtutis, quam ut solum sufficiat ad conceptum: quoniam frigidius est virili."

4. Castro, *De universa mulierum medicina* (Hamburg, 1603), pars 1, lib. 1, c. 3 (p. 28). There are other (and revised) eds. of 1617, 1628, 1644, and 1662.

5. Ian Maclean, *The Renaissance Notion of Woman: A Study in the Fortunes of Scholasticism and Medieval Science in European Intellectual Life* (Cambridge: Cambridge University Press, 1985), p. 29. On the larger problem (in terms of social construction) of changing attributions of abilities and values to males and females, see Thomas Laqueur, *Making Sex: Body and Gender from the Greeks to Freud* (Cambridge, Mass.: Harvard University Press, 1990).

6. Rodrigo a Castro, *De universa mulierum medicina,* pars 1, lib. 1, c. 6 (1603 ed., vols. 1, 12): ". . . hinc colligas, vulgatis illis gynaeciorum tribus voluminibus una cum praestanti doctrina, similes fabellas et prodigiosa multa figmenta contineri, quae facile possint tyronibus fucum facere." Borrowed from Maclean, *The Renaissance Notion of Women,* p. 29.

7. Castro, *De universa mulierum medicina,* pars 1, lib. 2, c. 3 (1642 ed.), p. 84.

8. Mercado, *Opera* (Frankfurt, 1620), vol. 1, p. 236: "Praeterquam quod nullus est vir adeo Veneris inexpertus, quod in concubitu non sentiat, penem foemineo semine spargi, et foeminas profusione calefieri: quod etiam mulieres ipsae in se experiuntur, quia ante virilis seminis susceptionem, sentiunt se humectari."

9. Jacques Dubois (Iacobus Sylvius), *De mensibus mulierum, et hominis generatione commentarius* in *Gynaeciorum sive de mulierum affectibus commentarii Graecorum, Latinorum, Barbarorum,* ed. Caspar Wolphius (Basel, 1587), pp. 306–07. On Dubois as "arch-Galenist of Paris," see Gerhard Baader, "Jacques Dubois as a Practitioner," in *The Medical Renaissance of the Sixteenth Century,* ed. A. Wear, R. K. French, and I. M. Lonie (Cambridge: Cambridge University Press, 1985), pp. 146–54.

10. See Audrey Eccles, *Obstetrics and Gynaecology in Tudor and Stuart England* (Kent, Ohio: Kent State University Press, 1982), pp. 49–50. But cf. also Patrica Crawford on English material: "Attitudes to Menstruation in Seventeenth-Century England," *Past and Present* 91 (1981): 47–73.

11. Mercuriale, *De hominis generatione,* in *Pisanae praelectiones* (Venice, 1597), p. 4; for the habits of the Gnostics, see p. 6.

12. *De medicorum principum historia* in *Opera omnia* (Lyon, 1642), vol. 1, p. 135 (misnumbered 235).

13. Ibid., pp. 266–67: "... in utere, qui est totius corporis cloaca, excrementorum sentina, ac receptaculum. Accedit innati caloris in foemineo sexu imbecillitas, putretudinis causas non repugnans."

14. See Bartolomeo Platina, *De honneste volupté* (Lyon, 1528), p. 4v.

15. Ilza Veith, *Hysteria: The History of a Disease* (Chicago and London: University of Chicago Press, 1965); *Witchcraft and Hysteria in Elizabethan London: Edward Jorden and the Mary Glover Case*, ed. with an introd. Michael MacDonald (London and New York: Tavistock/Routledge, 1991); Sander Gilman, Helen King, Roy Porter, George Rousseau, and Elaine Showalter, *Hysteria Beyond Freud* (Berkeley and Los Angeles: University of California Press, 1993). For the modern period, see Elaine Showalter, *The Female Malady: Women, Madness, and English Culture 1830–1980* (New York: Pantheon, 1985).

16. See my essay, "Burton's Use of *praeteritio* in Discussing Same-Sex Relationships," in *Renaissance Discourses of Desire*, ed. C. J. Summers and T. L. Pebworth (Columbia, MO. and London: University of Missouri Press, 1993), pp. 159–78.

17. Peter Foreest, *Observationum et curationum medicinalium libri*, vol. 28 (*De mulierum morbis*), observatio 26 (Lugd. Bat., 1599), pp. 151–53: "Vidua annum 44 agens, soror Laurentii Athenarii, Pastoris in pago Soechtwouda dicto, praeceptoris mei in iuventute, quae quidem Alcmariae habitabat prope gruem, anno 1546 mense Maio, gravissima uteri suffocatione laborabat. Cumque pro mortua haberetur, et quasi syncope afficeretur, subito ad eam vocatus fui. Erat autem suffocatio es semine retento. Mulierculae praesentes faciem vino aspergebant, naresque ac tempora oblinebant, putantes hoc modo illam posse a syncope excitari; sed hoc modo malum magis augebant . . . quamobrem ego hic ut ab irroratione tum aspersione ac frictione vini abstinerent iussi; et ut proprios pilas combustos olfaceret (cum plumae perdicis ad manum non essent) eosque pro odoratu continuo naribus admovebam; tum frictiones dolorosas pedum adhibebam, praecipue sub volis cum sale et aceto fortiter fricando: sua enim acuitate et punctione (eodem Grado teste) convertunt superfluitates ad inferiora, et excitant a paroxismo. Adhibebamus quoque ligaturas fortes circa coxas, modo relaxando, modo constringendo. Nam haec omnia cum laborem inferunt, etiam deturbant materiam ad inferiora, et inhibent ascensum vaporum ad superiora. Dum haec fiunt, necessitate urgent, obstetricem accersiri iussimus, ut intus fricando cum digito muliebria sequenti oleo inungeret. . . . Atque hoc modo praeter spem a paroxysmo excitata est. Talis autem titillatio cum digito ab omnibus Medicis, ut Galeno ac Avic. tum aliis, commendatur; praecipue in viduis et caste viventibus, ac monialibus, ut asserit Gradus: minus tamen iunioribus, et elocandis, vel maritum habentibus; cum excellentius remedium sit viro copulentur. Id tamen non nisi re valde urgente, aliis praesidiis non iuvantibus faciendum duco."

18. Corbeius, *Gynaeceium* (Frankfurt, 1620).

19. Giovanni Matteo da Grado, *Praxis in nonum Almansoris* (Lyon, 1527), fol. 454v.

20. Foreest, *Observationem*, vol. 28, p. 153: "Impudicum quoque consilium illud est cuiusdam mulierculae, ut pili pudendi vellicentur, quo suffocatae ad se redeant. Id quidem factum a chirurgo nimis impudenter dum famula quaedam subito suffocata solo prostata iaceret, multis praeterea in cubiculo existentibus, vidimus; et illa mox cum verecundia excitata ridentibus aliis, discessit, sanata."

21. Galen, *On the Affected Parts*, trans. Rudolph E. Siegel (Basel: Karger, 1976), p. 185; Kuehn ed., vol. 8, p. 420.

22. Abraham Zacuto, *De historia principum medicorum*, lib. 3, hist. 9, in *Opera omnia* (Lyon, 1642), vol. 1, p. 468.

23. Zacuto, *De praxi medica libri tres* (Amsterdam, 1634), lib. 2, observatio 85, p. 208: "Num autem ex hac occasione liceat medico timenti Deum, sopitis pariter cunctis sensibus, et una obolita respiratione, in foeminis quasi animam agentibus, seu in maximo vitae periculo constitutis veneficum illud semen foras ab utero, titillationibus, et frictionibus partium obscoenarum elidere...."

24. Castro, *De universa mulierum medicina*, pars 2, lib. 2, c. 1 (1603 ed., p. 102): "Tunc (si fieri id sine scelere possit) obstetrix collum uteri confricet digitis ... ut irritatus crassus humor, qui in utere haeret, provocetur, et calefactus excernatur."

25. Ibid., p. 108: "An liceat frictione facta in pudendo semen prolicere sapientibus discutiendum relinquo, advertens semen, quod eo tempore excernitur, prolificum iam non esse, sed venenatum, ac corporis excrementum inutile, et multorum malorum, saepe etiam mortis causam, adhaec foeminis invitis, aut saltem non consentientibus excerni."

26. *Gynaeciorum, hoc est de mulierum tum aliis, tum gravidarum, parientium, et puerperarum affectibus et morbis, Libri veterum ac recentiorum*, ed. Hans Kaspar Wolf (Basel, 1566). The passage from Dubois (Sylvius), from his chapter, "De uteri suffocatione et perversione," is on col. 833. The "arch-Galenist of Paris" is Baader's phrase, see fn. 9.

27. *Gynaeciorum sive de mulierum morbis*, ed. Israel Spach and Caspar Bauhin (Strassburg, 1597). Albertino Bottoni, *De morbis muliebribus* in c. 39, "De praefocatione matricis," with reference to Galen, and c. 46, "De pharmaca" (p. 375); Girolamo Mercuriale, *De morbis muliebribus*, lib. 4, c. 22, "De uteri praefocatione" (p. 302).

28. Luis Mercado, *De mulierum affectionibus libri quatuor*, lib. 2, c. 3 "De uteri strangulatione": "Sed cavere hac re oportet a titillationibus quas multi consulunt in partibus pudendis fieri, etiam si foeminas ob id levari excreto semine conspiciamus; nam scimus non licere medico christiano." In *Gynaeciorum sive de mulierum morbis*, ed. Spach and Bauhin, p. 892. Mercado's book was first published at Valladolid in 1579.

29. Ranchin, *Tractatus de morbis virginum*, sect. 3, c. 2 in *Opuscula medica* (Lyon, 1627), p. 423: "Gravis sane maximique momenti est proposita difficultas; an scilicet liceat confricare mulieres, seu contrectare earum naturalia in paroxismo hysterico. Qui laudant, confrictionem, authorithatibus, et rationibus non carent. Primo Galenus historiam proponit cuiusdam viduae, quae restituta fuit immisso digito ab obstetrice in uterum, atque effuso semine: unde iam invaluit consuetudo, ut pleraeque artificiosis instrumentis excavatis, et penis virilis formam referentibus utantur ad excitandam pollutionem voluntariam, et ad praecavenda hysterica symptomata. Secundo Avicenna mandat, ut obstetrices digitum vulvae immittant, atque fricent diligenter, ut ita seminalis materia excernatur."

30. Ibid.: "Unde apparet eiusmodi frictionem veneris vicem gerere, quam conferre iam probatum fuit; ac proinde inhumanum esse remedii istius salutaris usum dissuadere concludunt. Nos tamen secundum Theologorum doctrinam eiusmodi frictionem, ut abominabilem damnandum censemus, potissimum in Virginibus, cum talis pollutio Virginitatem corrumpat."

31. Ibid., p. 432: "Quod autem ad mulieres spectat, earum conscientiae remedii praxim committimus, cum respectus divini praecepti suadere, ac consulere Medicis Christianis non patiatur."

32. Moxius, *De methodo medendi per venae sectionem morbos muliebres acutos* (Geneva, 1612), p. 502: "Res sane difficilis et ardua, que multorum animos hactenus contorsit." On Moxius (or Moix), see Antonio Hernández Morejón, *Historia bibliográfica de la medicina española*, vol. 5 (Madrid, 1846), pp. 29–30.

33. Galen, *De locis affectis*, 6, c. 5; Kuehn ed., vol. 8, p. 418.

34. Moxius, *De methedo medendi*, p. 508: "Haec res ita difficilis est in actuosa Medicina, quod nulla altera, meo iudicio, difficilior occurrat: quia omnes Theologi conveniunt semine existente optimo, sola peccante quantitate nefas ulla ratione directe elidere."

35. Ibid. See Thomas Sanchez (1550–1610), *Disputationes de sancto matrimonii sacramento*, 3 vols. (Antverp, 1607), tom. 3, lib. 9, disp. 17, num. 19, p. 678 (2d count); the first ed. appears to be of 1602–05.

36. Ibid., p. 509: "Tertio confirmatur, quia licet cuique verenda refricare ad sedandum pruritum: licet itidem et chirurgis eadem verenda ostendere, ut morbis medeantur, clausas etiam aperiant, licet inde praeter intentionem sequatur pollutio."

37. Ibid.: "oppositam sententiam, seu tutiorem tenent Theologi plurimi, ac sane gravissimi quos consului, antequam ad nostras manus pervenisset opus Thomae Sanchez."

38. Ibid., p. 510: ". . . saltem quasi certo exponemus nos huic periculo, ob partium obscoenarum fricationem, et seminis a vesiculis illis abiunctionem; ut viduae illi Galenus contigisse scribit."

39. Ibid., 511: ". . . tamen exponemus nos huic periculo, et aeque tunc nobis imperantibus."

40. Sanchez, *Disputationes*, tom. 3, lib. 7, disp. 113, num. 21 (1607 ed.), pp. 439–40 (2d count).

41. For some examples of warnings against the physician's libidinous involvement, see Codronchi's warnings not to exploit situations with sick women and *molles adolescentes*, *De Christiana ac tuta medendi ratione*, (Ferrara, 1591), p. 108 (and his entire c. 36), as well as commentaries to the Hippocratic oath, which calls all persons belonging to the household of the patient off limits to the physician.

42. See ibid., lib. 1, c. 21 on *suffocatio ex redundante vel retento semine* and particularly p. 63: ". . . ut mea sert sententia difficilis solutionis, cum de hac

re peculiariter nihil quidquam ab aliquo scriptore, Summista potissimum literis mandatum ad huc invenerim."

43. Ibid., pp. 63–64: "Olim ego arbitratus fueram, si medico certum sit, et exploratum; hystericam adeo a sensibus destitutam fuisse; ut ex huiusmodi operatione nullam delectationis, aut voluptatis titillationem percipere posset, in manifestoque salutis discrimine versaretur, bono fine considerato, nulloque scandalo orituro tale praesidium posse tolerari."

44. Sennert, *Practica medica* (Paris, 1633), vol. 4, part. 2, sec. 3, chap. 4, p. 232: "a Christiano Medico susdenda non videatur." On Sennert, see Wolfgang-Uwe Eckart, "Grundlagen des medizinisch-wissenschaftlichen Erkennens bei Daniel Sennert (1572–1637) untersucht an seiner Schrift *De Chymicorum liber*," M.D. diss. (Universität Münster, 1978). Also Allen G. Debus, "Guintherius, Libavius and Sennert: The Chemical Compromise in Early Modern Medicine," in *Science, Medicine and Society in the Renaissance: Essays to Honor Walter Pagel*, ed. Allen G. Debus (London: Heinemann, 1972), vol. 1, pp. 151–65; and Peter H. Niebyl, "Sennert, Van Helmont and Medical Ontology," *Bulletin of the History of Medicine* 45 (1971): 115–37.

45. Eccles, *Obstetrics and Gynaecology in Tudor and Stuart England*, p. 79. Eccles is referring to the parenthetical comment that the English editors and translators inserted in their version of Lazare Rivière's sentence rejecting on moral grounds the cure by the midwife's titillation. In their editorial comment, they call their author "a silly superstitious Papist." See Nicholas Culpeper, Abdiah Cole, and William Rowland, *The Practice of Physick. Being chiefly a Translation of the Works of Lazarus Reverius* (London, 1672), vol. 1, pp. 427–28: "But seeing that [i.e. the rubbing and tickling by the midwife] cannot be done without wickedness (understand by a silly superstitious Papist, that counts it a meritorious good work to burn Mother and Child in her Womb alive, as at Jersey, and wickedness to free a sick Body of a little offensive Humor), a Christian Physician must never prescribe the same." See also James Primrose, *De morbis mulierum* (Rotterdam, 1655), p. 218. After describing the manipulation, Primrose says: "Verum an id liceat facere, & sic naturam ad semen expellendum irritare, Theologorum est inquirere. Non absurdè creditur id licere, quia tunc semen foeminis invitis, minimèque consentientibus excernitur, estque eiusmodi semen minimèque prolificum, sed venenum corporis, non solum inutile, sed etiam noxium excrementum. . . ."

46. Cortesi, *Miscellaneorum medicinalium decades* (Messina, 1625), p. 813. Since Moxius's work, to which Cortesi is responding, did not appear until 1612, A. de Ferrari appears to be wrong when surmising that the *Decades* were still written during Cortesi's period at Bologna, i.e. before 1599. See *Dizionario biográfico degli Italiani*, vol. 29 (Rome, 1983), p. 764.

47. Cortesi, *Decades*, p. 809: "Mihi, antequam rem attingam, opus est demonstrare determinationem quaesiti huius non pertinere ad Theologos, quorum consilium Moxius voluisse inquit, sed esse merum Medicorum negotium, aut saltem id, quod statuunt Theologi, pendere ex re medica."

48. Ibid., p. 815: "Utrum illa materia in muliebribus testibus sit semen, an excrementum, ut voluit Arist. alterius est negotii. . . ."

49. Ibid., p. 816: "Verum aliud est considerare semen putrefactum in cavitate uteri, quod nunquam emitti potest cum delectatione, et voluptate; et alius est loqui de semine mulieris contento in vasis spermaticis, praecipue in testibus, unde emittitur saepissime cum delectatione."

50. Ibid., p. 817: ". . . sive in uteri spatio nata, sive aliunde fluentia per apertam uteri cervicem in subiectam. . . ."

51. Ibid., p. 818: "Sed turpius quidem mea opinione Moxius erravit, qui Medicus est, praesuponens huiusmodi casum . . . ad liberandam mulierem iam animam agentem oportere effluxum seminis procurare."

52. Galen, On the Affected Parts, trans. R. E. Siegel (Basel: Karger, 1976), pp. 184–85 (bk. 6, chap. 5, ed. Littré, vol. 8, p. 419).

53. Zacuto, De medicorum principum historia in Opera omnia, vol. 1, p. 470.

54. Louis Duret (1527–1586), Commentary in Jacques Houllier, Opera omnia practica L. Dureti annotationibus (Geneva, 1623), p. 515: "At mulier quaevis, quia in otio degit, et corpus habet dysdiaphoreton si Venerem non exerceat, salubriter vivere nequit."

55. Ibid., p. 514: "quod colligitur ex comment. ad sent, 4 sect. 3 lib 3 Edid. sub finem."

56. Galen, On the Affected Parts, trans. Siegel, p. 197 (ed. Littre, vol. 8, pp. 450–51).

57. Zacuto, Opera omnia, vol. 1, p. 470: "Sed quomodo Galenus hunc vocaverit continentissimum, si scortum non expectans, manu propria semen excernens necessitati satisfecit?"

58. Ludovico Ricchieri, Lectionum antiquarum libri xxx (Basel 1542), lib. 20, c. 14, p. 775: "Lydiorum porro illud etiamnum peculiare, meridianis horis turpiter manibus indicere Talassionem, ut fieret sine foemina mariti."

59. Castro, De universa mulierum medicina, pars 2, lib. 1, c. 15 (1603 ed.), p. 69.

60. Ibid.: "Haec doctis duntaxat scripta velim, plane omittenda, si quis hanc praxin vernaculo transferat sermone, ne levioribus ingeniiis, et depravatis mentibus foedissimi sceleris via monstretur. Atque idcirco scholium hoc, quoad fieri potuit contraxi, non tam de inopia, aut sterilitate materiae, quam de pudoris magnitudine."

61. Lloyd DeMause, "The Evolution of Childhood," in The History of Childhood: The Untold Story of Child Abuse (New York: Pedrick, 1988): p. 48; 1st ed., 1974.

62. Bruce R. Smith, Homosexual Desire in Shakespeare's England: A Cultural Poetics (Chicago and London: University of Chicago Press, 1991), p. 49.

63. Zacuto, Opera omnia, vol. 1, p. 31 (lib. 1, hist. 19).

64. Tomás Rodriguez da Veiga, In Claudii Galeni libros De locis affectis (Antverp, 1566), p. 331. On the fortunes of Galenism, see Owsei Temkin, Galenism: Rise and Decline of a Medical Philosophy (Ithaca, N.Y., and New York: Cornell University Press, 1973).

65. Moxius, De methodo medendi, pp. 506–07: "Verum lethaliores multo affectus censet, quos parat semen corruptum, utique pariter sexui familiares.

Nam et viris accidere declarat illud Angeli Politiani de Michaele Verino epigramma, Sola Venus. . . ."

66. Daniel Sennert, *Epitome institutionum medicinae*, lib. 4, part. 1, c. 8 (Patavia, 1644), p. 343: "Semen impestive retentum corporis gravitatem, et torporem inducit, et si corrumpatur gravissima accidentia excitat; quae Venere omnia evitare licet. Verum sit ea tempestiva, et legitima. Neque enim sanitatis conservandae gratia tentare aliquid opus est, quod legibus divinis sit contrarium; Creatorque homini tantum hac in re indulsit, quantum ad omnia, quae sanitati obesse possunt, evitanda est necessarium."

67. Hans Peter Duerr, *Der Mythos vom Zivilisationsprozess*, 2 vols. 1: *Nacktheit und Scham* (Frankfurt: Suhrkamp, 1988–90); vol. 2: *Intimität* (Frankfurt: Suhrkamp, 1990).

68. Fallopius, *De decoratione*, *Opera omnia* (Frankfurt, 1600), vol. 2, pp. 338–39: "Ego moneo parentes, ut studeant in aetate infantili, ut magnificetur membrum puerorum."

69. Ibid., p. 339: "His rationibus, per transversam fricando, extendimus priapum. Fit etiam hoc calefacientibus, ut testaignea accepta intra crura, vel pannis calidis. Sed observate, ut statim quum concidit pudendum, erigatis, vel pannis calidis, vel alio calido; nam hoc iuvat pueris, et etiam consistentibus. Sed advertant imbecilles, non abundantes copia spirituum, ne extensa vasa spiritu implere non possint. Hoc autem fiet per medicamenta proposita a practicis."

70. Duerr, *Der Mythos vom Zivilisationsprozess*, vol. 1, *Nacktheit und Scham* (1988), p. 208.

71. Fallopius, *Opera Omnia*, vol. 2, p. 339: "Hoc quod dico, et quod in posterum dicturus sum, necessitate generationis coactus assero, non quod quid contra legem aut contra bonos mores promulgare audeam."

72. Ibid., p. 342.

73. Ibid., p. 340: "Si autem quaeratur, Cur Deus altissimus in populo electo instituit, ut afferetur praeputium, causae sunt eternae, et positae in mente Altissimi quas non oportet dicere in profanis scholis."

74. Ibid., p. 341.

75. Ibid., pp. 341–42.

76. Johann Heinrich Meibom, (1590–1655), *A Treatise of the Use of Flogging in Venereal Affairs: Also of the Office of the Loins and Reins* (London, 1718). This is a translation of Thomas Bartholin and Johann Heinrich Meibom, *De usu flagrorum in re medica et venerea* (Frankfurt, 1670), which in addition to the original letter by Johann Heinrich Meibom includes a somewhat pedantic letter, dated 1669, by Bartholin on the same subject and a response to it by the physician Heinrich Meibom, son of Johann Heinrich. Since Bartholin's letter is adorned with a quotation from Juvenal, a reference to the Roman Lupercalia ("Nudus . . . pulset puellas") and allusion to the pleasure women take in being beaten, it would seem that at the time when the elaborate physiology Meibom had drawn upon to make his point was proven to be old-fashioned and faulty, publishers began to market Meibom's letter as pornography. I have not seen the first edition (mentioned by Claude Mercier in his edition of the letter [Paris, 1792], in his "avis de l'éditeur"), but have used the edition

of Leiden, 1643. The NLM also has an edition called "editio secunda" on the title page and assigned to 1650, not listed by Mercier. The edition printed as of "London, 1665" is (according to Mercier) of Paris, 1757. The English translation of 1718 was redone in modern spelling as John Henry Meibomius, *On the Use of Flogging in Venereal Affairs* (Chester, Pa.: Import Publishing Co., 1961), however, with a date for the letter (1659) that must be erroneous, since it is after the author's death.

77. On the other hand, the engraving in Mercier's ed. (Paris, 1792), showing several scantily dressed young women surrounding a baby/Cupid, whose bottom one of the women is spanking, is not only coy but misleading.

78. In his commentary on the Hippocratic oath, Meibom gives his version of a history of same-sex relationships, which he sharply condemns: *Horkos, sive jusjurandum* (Leiden, 1643), pp. 181–85. For a contemporary condemnation of female same-sex relationships in a work that claims to address medical questions, see Heinrich Kornmann, *Sybyla Tryg Andriana, seu De Virginitate, virginum statu et iure tractatus* (Frankfurt, 1610). Chapter 48, entitled "Qua poena puniantur virgines fricantes se?" threatens young women with death by fire. What is to be understood by *fricatio* is deliberately left obscure lest young women be tempted to the practice: "Quo vero modo illa fricatio fiat, tacere quam exprimere melius est, ne virginibus memoria et cogitatio eius rei daretur" (pp. 135–36).

79. Meibom, *Horkos, sive Jusjurandum.*

80. *De flagrorum usu*, p. 48 (1643 ed.). "Nullus vetabo."

81. Ibid.: *crimen invidentiae.*

82. Green, "Women's Medical Practice and Health Care in Medieval Europe," *Signs* 14 (1989): 434–73.

83. Critique of the limited knowledge of the women practicing health care is frequent with the academically trained physicians I am reviewing, and I agree with Monica Green's desiratum that "the question of rivalry between medical practioners could be addressed with far greater nuance" (Ibid., p. 456). But her example (from Guainerio through Helen Lemay), which is meant to show that he sets himself off economically from those women (he uses the ungendered word "vulgares") by more expensive prescriptions, in this case using asafetida and castoreum rather than burnt feathers to create foul odors, needs to be balanced by the fact that Guainerio elsewhere also suggests using *stercor thauri sive bovis*, i.e. bullshit, for the same medical purpose. See Helen R. Lemay, "Anthonius Guainerius and Medieval Gynecology," in *Women of the Medieval World: Essays in Honor of John H. Munday*, ed. Julius Kirshner and Suzanne F. Wemple (Oxford and New York: Blackwell, 1985), p. 327.

84. See Owsei Temkin, *Galenism: Rise and Decline of a Medical Philosophy*, particularly p. 161; and Nancy G. Siraisi, *Avicenna in Renaissance Italy: The Canon and Medical Teaching in Italian Universities after 1500* (Princeton, N.J.: Princeton University Press, 1987). Siraisi shows that through the Renaissance medicine tended to be taught by commentary. While her emphasis is on the longevity of the *Canon* (which, particularly in Roman Catholic Europe, had in medical education survived the opposition of Galenic humanists), she also

recognizes its decline after 1620, together with "the gradual replacement of Aristotelian philosophy and Galenic physiology" (pp. 84 and 120 respectively).

85. The edition printed at Brescia, 1624, however, still has the old paragraph 19 (vol. 3, p. 224)!

86. Lemay, "Anthonius Guainerius," p. 323.

87. Guainerio, *Tractatus de matricibus*, in *Opera omnia* (Pavia, 1481, f. x4rb): "Obstetrix deinde os vulve perungat iniunctumque digitum si corrupta fuerit quanto plus poterit immitat matricis collum . . ."; from Lemay, "Anthonius Guainerius," p. 323.

88. Ranchin, *Tractatus de morborum virginum*, p. 423: "Nos tamen secundum theologorum doctrinam eius modi frictionem, ut abominabilem damnandam censemus, potissimum in Virginibus, cum talis pollutio Virginitatem corrumpat."

89. See my essay, "'That Matter Which Ought Not To Be Heard Of': Homophobic Slurs in Renaissance Cultural Politics," *Journal of Homosexuality* 26 (1994): 41–75.

6

Renaissance Moralizing about Syphilis and Prevention

While the problems of removing male and female seed have received little attention by modern historians of medicine or of anthropology, the history of venereal disease—more specifically, the *morbus Gallicus* or syphilis—has been the focus of considerable interest. Modern discussions include the following questions: Was the *morbus Gallicus* a new disease or not? Why did it spread so quickly at the end of the fifteenth century? How and why did cures shift during the Renaissance (for instance, from mercury to guaiacum or *lignum Indicum*)? To what extent did the difficulty or even impossibility of integrating the disease into humoral medicine contribute to that system's demise? All these questions are of only peripheral interest in my context, for my focus is the moral interpretation of the disease (most notably as *flagellum Dei* or punishment of God), and moral issues relating to its prevention. On the one hand, my topic is an aspect of the larger nexus between sin and pathology as discussed by Paul Diepgen for the Middle Ages; on the other hand, through its multinational scope, it complements other actual or possible approaches to the moral interpretation of syphilis, for example: Owsei Temkin's emphasis on the difference between the three virulent decades immediately after the disease first appeared, when (as he claims) it was not generally recognized as a venereal disease, and the period after 1520 or 1530, when the connection was generally made; Temkin's claim that the gentler guaiacum therapy was reserved for the nobility, while the common people were subjected to the torture of mercury "for the atonement of their sins"; and, finally, the distinction between accounts of syphilis by writers who revealed themselves as sufferers from the disease (the German nobleman von Hutten, the Spanish priest Francisco Delgardo, the German secretary to Maximilian I, Joseph Grünpeck, perhaps even the artist Benvenuto Cellini) and accounts by writers not suffering from it, since one may assume that having or not having syphilis would color a person's moral interpretations of the disease.

Undoubtedly Anthony Grafton is correct when he says in a recent review of Renaissance writings on syphilis that "the most striking feature of this literature is, indeed, the power of existing explanations, beliefs, and social attitudes, many of them traditional, to incorporate the experience."[1] My interest is both more general and more precise. Except for occasional references to von Hutten or an interpretation by a moral theologian, I deal with works by surgeons or physicians. Restricting my focus to the Renaissance allows me to cross national and geographic borders with the hope of arriving at some tentative comparisons. To what extent, in different parts of Europe, was this particular disease not considered accidental but a deserved punishment for individuals or groups (or nations)? How did moral tenets about syphilis influence medical teaching about prevention? Who were the intended readers of these books, most of which were written in Latin? How did women figure in the early construction of this disease, both as infectors and as healers?

If some English writers are discussed here first, this is not to suggest that theirs were in any way central and innovative minds in diagnosing and curing the disease—in fact, of the roughly one hundred works that Lipenius lists on the subject a few decades after the end of the period of my interest,[2] none appears to have been by an English author. I am dealing with only one facet of a complex of problems relating to the disease, however—moral interpretation; and there can be no question that in the field of medical ethics, what was printed in English soon came to be important.

Some English Syphilographers

As is well known, most Renaissance writers considered syphilis a new disease, although they did not necessarily believe that it had been imported from America by Christopher Columbus's sailors. In his famous treatise celebrating what he thought was an effective remedy, Ulrich von Hutten found that its recent (though not explicitly American) origin was the only matter relating to it that the physicians of his time could agree upon, and this statement appears generally true although not disinterested, since Hutten had set out to praise the effectiveness of the "Indian wood." (Before and after von Hutten, however, there were some dissenters from this view, of whom Nicolò Leoniceno [1428–1524] was one of the best known.)[3] In any case, in his *Methode of Phisicke*, the Englishman Philip Barrough (fl. 1590) assumes the American origin as a standard element of medical history in his account, to which he gives an anti-Catholic moral-political slant:

> First, the Spaniardes borrowed it of the Indians, and brought it home in stead of their gold, and afterward *Charles* the fift Emperour of Rome, who was a man of great power, and delighted much in shedding of bloud, spared neither man, woman, nor child; insomuch that he spoiled a great part of Italy, and subdued the dukedom of Millan, with great hurt, ruine and spoile, to all the commonwealth of Florence: and at the last he came to Rome and Naples, with his whole hoast, spoyling all as he went with great cruelty: and for his hire, this disease began first to show it selfe plentifully among his people, and specially because his soldiers were much given to venery.[4]

Barrough's account is clearly spiked: there is the ironic switching of disease for expected gold; and rather than heading the Holy Roman Empire, Charles is the Emperor of Rome, a city that to Elizabethans connotes the home of the Antichrist. (In later editions, as for instance, the sixth edition [1624], the same passage reads "Charles the eight, King of France.") Of course such anti-Roman sentiment (and the link with syphilis) was not limited to England but expressed in other Protestant countries as well. Toward the end of the seventeenth century, the Dutch physician Stephen Blankaart (1650–1702) records a malicious anagram using the first letters of "Spanische Pocken Quälen Rom" (Spanish pocks torture Rome): S P Q R, conventionally standing for *Senatus Populusque Romanus*.[5] Barrough makes Charles V a sadist enjoying destruction. The outbreak of the disease in his army at Naples is ironically presented as the reward or pay ("hire") specifically for him, for his cruelty, and generally, for his soldiers for being "much given to venery." Providential history thus has been using the disease for a purpose, as he makes even clearer when he continues: "The frenchmen at that siege got the buttons of Naples (as we terme them) which does much annoy them at this day. But the first finding of this grievous sicknesse, was brought into Spaine, by *Columbus* at his coming home, so that all Christendome may curse the Emperour and *Columbus*." Thus, at the time when a major encounter with Spain was already looming (the first edition of the book is of 1583), Barrough sees the disease as a deserved curse on everything the Elizabethans hate: the Emperor, Rome, and the Spanish. According to Barrough:

> Then *Columbus* travelled again, and brought with him little gold, but all his men were well infected with this griefe: insomuch that the Physitions in those daies did not knowe what to make of the griefe, nor how to helpe the people. So for want of knowledge many were spoiled. After (as I told you before of the Siege of Naples) the Spaniards for friendship they bare to the Frenchmen, sent to them of their curtizans infected with this griefe, minding to let them have some of their iewels, which they brought out of the Indian countrey. The Frenchmen (not knowing their kind hearts) fell in love with them, and (being ravished with their beauty) dealt with them, to their great cost and trouble to this day. Now to the variety of names: First, the Italians call it *Morbus Gallicus*, and some call it *Variolam Gallicam*, because it first appeared among the Frenchmen at the siege before named. The French call it *Scabiem Hispanicam*, because the Spaniards first brought it out of the Indies. The Germans call it *Menium*, why they should term it so, I know not well, unless *Menium* doe signifie the privy parts infected with this disease. Some of them call it also *Scabiem Hispanicam*. In Spaine they name it *Morbum Neapolitanum*, the cause I told you before . . . and we in our countrey call it the French disease. But however it bee called it skilleth not, so that we knowe how to helpe it, which I minde to declare hereafter by Gods grace. (p. 362)

Although this account seems to contain straightforward and even commonplace information, it is not as innocent as it may first appear: there is the ironic exchange or *commercium* of Columbus bringing infection instead of the expected gold; the ironic "friendship" of the Spaniards (really their malice of sending infected women to the French); the wordplay in "jewels" (those about which they are misers versus those metaphorical jewels with which they are generous, i.e their genitals or even their sores or "buttons") and in the Frenchmen's "knowing" the Spaniards' kind hearts (which is both knowing and not knowing and leads to another kind of knowing, their "dealing" with the women). I cannot tell whether Barrough entirely invented these malicious interpretations. Curiously, the more topically reported acts of harming the opponent during these campaigns

are more specific than the ones narrated by the English physician
(and are usually adduced as an alternative to the "American hypothesis" to explain the sudden emergence of the disease, thus serving a
specific medical rather than a moral-political purpose): they include
the report that the Spanish poisoned the water for the French troops
(Gabriele Falloppio) or that they added the blood of lepers to the
wine of the French (David Planis Campi).[6]

The philological material then added by Barrough is also standard in most Renaissance works on syphilis. Some of the comments
are appropriately tentative, as on the Germans' reported name for the
illness, information that may derive from Ulrich von Hutten's well-
known work on syphilis and its cure.[7] Displaying the name of something is of course a traditional rhetorical strategy dating from the time
when the etymology of a word (as even the etymology of *etymology*
indicates) was thought to reveal some part of the "truth" of what it
named. Even with Barrough's final disclaimer that "however it bee
called it skilleth not," the survey of names (except for some debatable
item like *menium* or, in a sentence I omitted, *pendendagra* [for
pudendagra?]) has the cumulative effect of validating the previously
given moralized history of the disease.

At least Barrough is straightforward and quite specific on cures
for the disease, unlike William Bullein (d. 1576) a couple of decades
before him, who prefaced his list of somewhat more cursory prescriptions with a harsh invective against what would have been a considerable segment of his most interested readership of this section: Bullein
said that his therapy was not intended for those who had contracted
the disease by their own fault—which amounts to an at least rhetorical refusal to treat them:

> Yet would I not, that any should fyshe for thys disease, or be
> bolde when he is bitten, to thynke hereby to be helped: but
> rather eschue the cause of thys infirmity and filthy, rotton, burn-
> ing of Harlots etc. As to fly from the Pestylence, or from a wylde
> fyre, for what is more to be abhorred, than a pocky, fylthy, stynk-
> ing Carcasse? But if through blynde Ignorance, sodayne chaunce
> etc. any gotten it: then do thus to be delivered from it.[8]

Like Bullein, who would not encourage anyone "to fyshe for thys
disease," Barrough has little to say about prevention. When he

touches on the topic, he addresses also those recovering from it, trying to prevent a relapse.

Typical of most writers on the subject, including the continental ones (some of whom he cites), Barrough's perspective is entirely male; he sees the infection as coming from women (usually prostitutes, but also infected nurses):

> Chiefly *Venus* must be shut out of the dore quite, especially while this decoction [guaiacum] is in giving. Some by committing this act but once in this cure have failed of remedy through the same. There be develish women desirous to be handled and dealt withall, who will beautifie themselves, to inflame mens hearts to lust towards them; abandon these your company, and thrust them out of the dores and house. (p. 373–74)

The male perspective is just as apparent in the work on syphilis by William Clowes the Elder (1540–1604), a surgeon who many times refers to his practical experience in dealing with the disease. Clowes's statement about transmission takes into account the fact that babies can receive the disease from a nurse or parent who is infected, but he makes no attempt to explain how women might contract it: "The sickness is sayed first to be engendred by the accompaning [*sic*] with unclene women, which although it be most commonly true, yet it is not alwayes so, not in all persons."[9]

Clowes's moralizing of the disease, although not any less pronounced than Barrough's, has different characteristics. In contrast to Barrough's manner of turning the history of the disease to nationalistic propaganda, Clowes's nationalism is turned inward, to stirring the English to recognizing their sins. At the same time the disease remains God's just punishment (as he says in the prefatory epistle): "Lues Venerea, the pestilent infection of filthie lust: a sickness verie loathsome, odious, troublesome, and dangerous. A notable testimonie of the iust wrath of God against that filthie sinne, which at this daie not onely infecteth Naples, Spaine, and France, but increaseth yet daily, spreading it self through Englande . . ." (sig. Aiii). He reports that, together with three other surgeons or physicians, he has in five years cured "one thousand and more" at the Hospital of St. Bartholomew (fol. 1^v), where in nine or ten years, on the average, every other patient asking for treatment "had the pockes" (fol. 2). Thus he speaks with authority when he claims that the medical problem of the disease (which to him is at least as much a moral problem) has become eminently and perhaps even primarily English: "The disease was never in mine opinion more rife among the *Indians, Neapolitans,* yea in *Italie, France,* or *Spaine,* then it is at this daye in the Realme in *England,* I praye God quickly deliver us from it, and remove from us that filthy sinne that breedeth, nurseth, and disperseth it" (fol. 1–1ᵛ).

With his aim of a moral reformation in England, Clowes reveals his Puritan leanings, which are also evident both in his analysis of the social origin of the disease and his proposal of a remedy: "The causes whereof, I see none so great as the licencious and beastly disorder of a great number of rogues, and vagabonds, the filthy lyfe of many leude and idle persons, both men and women, about the Citie of London" (fol. 1ᵛ). Social and moral disorder go together and, in this case, breed disease. That Clowes needs to add the admission that in these ale-houses among the "dis-ordered persons, some other of better disposition, are many times infected," is reverse proof that for him the lower class and moral depravity go essentially together.

It is consistent with Clowes's generally moralized view of syphilis that in his advice about prevention of the disease a moral sense (loathing of sin) is invoked in the interest of avoidance of infection.

> And foreasmuch as the best avoiding and curing of everie disease, consisteth in shunning and removing the cause thereof, I wish all men generally, especially those which be infected, to loathe, detest, hate, and abhorre that striking sinne that is the original cause of this infection, and to praie earnestly to God the heavenlie Physition and Chirurgeon, for his gratious assistance to the perfect amendment of life, the most safest and surest waie to remove it. (Aiii–Aiiiᵛ)

While the opening clause of this sentence draws on a medical commonplace, the passage actually argues that there is a link between this sin and sickness or, more specifically, that disease is but a manifestation of sin, and that hence avoidance of sin, a moral sense, is the most powerful motivation in taking care of one's health. By pointing to sin as "the original cause of this infection," he may also be invoking associations with original sin.

Of course, in that period a preacher's striking that note would hardly be noteworthy.[10] Similar uses of disease, particularly the French disease, but also of the plague, could be demonstrated in dozens of writings belonging to various religious genres written by persons belonging to groups we now call "Puritans." Thus George Wither (1588–1667) devotes the entire second canto of his long poem *Britain's Remembrancer* to demonstrating that the reason for the plague is God's "fury." (Perhaps significantly, the pestilence was "discover'd at / A Frenchmans house without the *Bishopgate*."[11]) But Wither is not a physician and therefore is beyond the scope of my topic, which is to surmise that the surgeon Clowes's sympathy with the Puritan cause led him to blend medical cure with moral regeneration. Clowes encourages the magistrate to assume a task both moral-religious and civic, namely to seek "correction and punishment of this filthie vice, as also the reformation of those places above mentioned" (fol. 1ᵛ). Indeed, the idea of prevention by moral reform is at the core of Clowes's publication.

He seems to be trying to discourage any prospective readers who might pick up his book in order to cure themselves or to reduce the chance of infection *without* changing their sexual habits: "And here I protest that the very cause that moved me to set forth this booke, is not to encourage those wretches that wallow in this sinne, to continue in their beastlie lyfe, hoping by this booke, or any other whatsoever, to be able to deliver themselves from this sicknesse" (fol. 2). Therefore it is understandable that one does not find in Clowes's book even the minimal advice on hygiene that by then had become standard in continental works on syphilis, namely that the male should wash his member carefully immediately after intercourse.

Of course Clowes was familiar with this and other recommended preventive measures through Almenar, Falloppio (whom he cites), and others. Clowes published a translation of Almenar's *Treatise on the French Pocks*, with a chapter (5) on prevention entitled, "What cautions must be observed to escape the French Pockes," in which the Spanish author recommends such cleansing as well as application of a certain powder to the penis after intercourse. Almenar (fl. 1500) also says that absolute prevention means abstention and avoidance of sin, but restrains his moral-theological zeal. Clowes translates: "They which are careful to escape the French Pockes, let them first escheve sinne. But because these things perteine to another Phisition, this shall be sufficient."[12] As we have seen in Clowes's own treatise, to call himself back from moral reform and leave that topic to the theologian would be inconsistent with the Puritan temperament of this Elizabethan physician.

Like Bullein and Barrough, Clowes is tight-lipped on prevention. In a general sense Theodor Rosebury is no doubt correct when he says that in the centuries after Shakespeare's death the subject of syphilis became shameful. He adds: "And English influence, beneficial, baneful, or whatever it may have been, ranged over the world."[13] But if we are willing to accept a writer's forthrightness about prevention as a litmus test, we will have to acknowledge that the English moral or moralizing tradition (which we may loosely call "puritan") goes much further back: to medical works decades before Shakespeare's death.

Writing on Prevention South of the Alps

Without retracing early continental writings about syphilis in detail, I can say confidently that the moral vision in them is not so pronounced and general as in England. In his treatise, written with the encouragement of Paul Ricius (or Paolo Ricci), professor of medicine at Padua, Ulrich von Hutten (not a physician and not a disinterested observer, since he had the disease) had already ridiculed priests for espousing moral views of syphilis as if they were revealed fact.[14] Particularly medical works in Italy (very numerous on this topic and diligently read in northern Europe) do not seem to be informed by the degree of moral conviction that gives some logical consistency to the English treatises but is also their limitation,[15] although even here an occasional moralizing strain attaches itself to the writing about this disease. After all, the fictional shepherd Syphilus of Fracastoro's famous epic, after whom the disease is named, receives the disease as punishment for having overturned the sun god's altars.

I begin with Gaspar Torrella of Valencia (1452–1520), who as the personal physician of Pope Alexander VI (and also of his notorious son Cesare Borgia) came to live at Rome, where he published his *Tractatus cum consiliis contra pudendagram seu morbum Gallicum* (1497). Sudhoff and Singer report that "[at] the beginning of his exposition Torrella speaks of the disease as due to the divine wrath and to the influence of the stars, the familiar *flagellum Dei* and the *constellatio corporum superiorum* of the Middle Ages."[16] Since this makes Torrella sound like a spiritual ancestor of Barrough and Clowes, we should examine the passage in question:

The astrologers say that this disease comes from the constellation of the higher bodies. For they say that the universal effect must be traced back to universal causes. Others say that it is God's punishment (*flagitium Dei*).[17]

Torrella here uses *dicunt* ("they say") three times, which has the effect of distancing him from the views reported—Sudhoff and Singer are imprecise if not misleading in this regard. Indeed, that this physician of the Borgias is quite secular in his sensibility (although he was rewarded with a bishopric) also speaks through his advice about prevention: primarily directing his advice at (supposedly celibate) clerics, he recommends that if one cannot entirely abstain from women, one ought at least to find those who are not infected.[18]

Like the Spaniard Almenar, Nicolò Massa (d. 1569), cited much more often in the Renaissance than Torrella, advises the male to wash his groin immediately after intercourse, and then supplies hints about how to recognize whether his female partner is infected.[19] Massa begins his book by pointing out that with many people the disease does not immediately affect the genital area and by giving some memorable examples of how the disease was transmitted without sexual intercourse (from nurse to infant and from infant to nurse). The effect of this account in which he speaks of infected patients aged three, six, and eleven, can only be to remove from the disease some of the moral opprobrium of promiscuity (Massa, pp. 14–15). At the same time there is still in Massa's work a general sense of religious boundedness within which cure is attempted, as he puts it, "with divine guidance (from which all good things derive)."[20]

From the second half of the sixteenth century, we have the account of Henri Estienne (1531–1598) about what struck him as he attended a medical lecture at the famous University of Padua. In the book into which Estienne incorporated his impressions, the outstanding philologist and committed Protestant argues in great detail that the modern world, notably the "popish" culture controlled by Rome, surpasses the ancient world in decadence. *La vérole* (syphilis) is grist for his mill, for he too interprets it as God's punishment for promiscuity, notably in Rome. In the absence of accounts by Protestant Englishmen about attending medical lectures on our subject in Italy, we may let Estienne's reaction stand for what some radical English Protestants might have experienced in Padua: "In fact, I remember well finding myself in Padua in a lecture by Falloppio, in which he promised his students that the following day he would teach them the means of womanizing to their heart's content without any fear of Mme. Vérole or any of her accoutrements."[21] After "finding himself" in the lecture of the famous professor—at least rhetorically a way of minimizing his responsibility for being there—and finding his moral sensibility offended, Estienne apparently did not return to hear the sequel of the lecture, and in any case that same moral sensibility would have forbidden him to communicate Falloppio's preventive means.

But fortunately we have Falloppio's *De morbo Gallico*, apparently a transcript made by a student of his lectures, which seems to bear out Estienne's recollection. In chapter 89, entitled, "About Preservation from the French Disease," Falloppio (1523–1562) says: "I would seem to have achieved nothing unless I taught you how someone who sees a most beautiful 'siren' and sleeps with her although she is infected can avoid the French disease. I have always thought that there should be a method of prevention so that ulcerations would not come about through transmission of this kind. But what is that method?"[22] Falloppio then expounds upon the careful cleaning of the male organ after intercourse, by the middle of the sixteenth century a standard recommendation for prevention (if concern with prevention can be considered "standard"). Realizing that cleansing may not always be successful in removing the infection from the susceptible glands, Faloppio is searching for some topical agent to apply to the penis strong enough to penetrate it and then extract and "vanquish" the infectious matter. "Thus I have looked for such a medication. But since we also have to think of the frame of mind of the prostitutes, we cannot bring with us ointments from home: therefore I have invented a small cloth, soaked in medication, that can easily be brought along if you have pants (*femoralia*) wide enough to carry your entire pharmacy with you."[23] Falloppio explains that after intercourse he expects his students to clean themselves and cover the penis with a cloth bag prepared to size and soaked several times in particular ointments. He says that he made the "experiment" on eleven hundred men and calls on God as witness that none of them became infected. Claude Quétel is factually correct but somewhat judgmental when he says: "In a sense, then, Fallopio's protective is a precursor of the 'French letter,' although it is not impossible that the Romans, a highly depraved people, had already adopted methods of this sort."[24]

The quoted sentences highlight Falloppio's secular and possibly amoral stance with respect to disease prevention. The encounter with the good-looking *sirena* that the physician wants to make "safe" is clearly imagined to be casual. His word for the woman invokes Homer's nefarious females whose attraction Ulysses was able to resist only by having himself tied to a mast, i.e. by total and enforced abstinence. The later reference to *meretrices* (prostitutes) disambiguates the matter further. What is extraordinary, however, is that such a secular stance coexists in this work with a moralized view of the origin of disease in general and of this disease in particular: "This is permanent and eternal dogma: that because of sin came death and because of failing, punishment. Thus it came about that God has punished our sins by diseases."[25] Falloppio reports in this context that the victorious Pompey in his triumph brought leprosy from Egypt to Rome. In turn, the Hebrews and Egyptians knew the *morbus elephanticus*, while it was unknown among the Italians, Gauls, and the Germanic tribes: that disease spread first to Rome and from there to other areas. The point of his historical digression is to show that graver sins (*maiora peccata*) called for new diseases in the past and continue to do so in the present. He fails to name these new diseases and by some form of *praeteritio* claims he is abstaining from a theological interpretation: "The cause of this I leave for the theologians to explain."[26] Nevertheless, as to "the most recent" disease, he himself gives a moral-theological reasoning and theodicy: "The newest disease is the one we are talking about and call the French disease, sent from God so that, made more cautious, we stop indulging in promiscuity and devote ourselves to the study of letters and all the other useful arts."[27] Although the perception of specific illnesses as God's punishment is not unusual in sixteenth-century writings, it would seem that Falloppio's ideas go a little beyond the commonplace in that he sees syphilis not merely as punishment for some "other" (of another nationality [England's foe, as in Barrough], or the incorrigibly promiscuous), but as a corrective to the sexual habits of all of "us," including himself.

It could be that by calling the link between disease and sin "dogma," Falloppio is not only removing it from the purview of the physician to that of the theologian, but that he is also taking it to some axiomatic realm within which for him argumentation does not have the same cogency as within the field of medicine. But I admit that this hypothesis may be circular, since I am brought to this explanation by the seeming contradiction between his theology and his medical advice, which I am trying to explain. The notion of syphilis as a means (even if divine) of correcting or controlling human sexual habits is at the borderline of entirely secular notions of health care: by all moral or theological accounts, it is a higher form of virtue to resist sin for the love of the good (or of God) than merely for the avoidance of infection. And in any case, like other medical writers on syphilis before and after him, Falloppio knows that even the innocent (for instance infants) get infected and, therefore, that the link between this illness and sin is inconsistent. To point up such difficulties is not to blame this distinguished physician for failing to express a believable theodicy in the face of disease (for one may doubt, with Albert Camus's characters in *The Plague*, whether such can be had), but to notice that Falloppio does not carry his analysis very far. And surely, if Falloppio's notion of correcting sexual habits by the threat of infection is almost secular, his medical advice to his students for prevention is entirely so. Thus his nexus between the new disease and sin on the one hand, and his notions of prevention on the other are not quite as contradictory as they may at first appear.

In Italy, Falloppio's method of safeguarding against syphilis entered the mainstream of writing about the disease. Thus, in his *Luis venereae perfectissimus tractatus* (Patavii, 1597), Ercole Sassonia (1551–1607) reports Falloppio's ideas at length and develops them even further (chap. 16: *De praeservatione*), although he shows a measure of skepticism in his warning that anyone living promiscuously may not escape the disease for long (fol. 10). Also, in Sassonia, there is no question that the elaborate passage instructing the reader about what lotions to use for cleansing and how to prepare the cloth that will enclose the male member after intercourse is intended for frequenters of prostitutes. Indeed the *index rerum et verborum* summarizes the subject as, "Remedies for those who use a prostitute, so that they may not be so easily infected by the disease."[28] Sassonia's skepticism may be fueled also by his recognition that *lues venerea*, which as infectious disease he considers to be of a "cause" or origin (*causa*) "dark, malicious, and hot" (fol. 1), can be transmitted by sharing cups and meals. As always in this context, *causa occulta* points to a cause that is dark in the sense of unknown (or inexplicable in the traditional Galenic system); particularly with this physician of a predominantly secular temperament, the word does not have the meaning of our *occult*. Any attempt on Sassonia's part at an inclusive moral interpretation of the disease is checked by his knowledge that innocent people (he specifically mentions midwives [fol. 2]) can be infected.

For Eustachio Rudio (1551–1611), a professor at Padua, the French disease has a similarly problematic position within Galenic medicine and is therefore included in his work *Dark and Poisonous Diseases*. In his chapter on prevention,[29] he also refers to Falloppio and elaborates on the prescriptions of the latter: the compress is to be

worn on the penis even *before* intercourse to fortify it against infection
(p. 191). Falloppio's recommendation for cleansing after the act, his
piece of cloth carefully prepared to enclose the penis, as well as his
bragging account of successes, are all reported in detail, although
Rudio recommends avoidance of prostitutes "and similar women" as
the safest prevention (p. 192; also p. 168).

Rudio's discussion of the disease and his recommendations for
prevention are possibly even more secularly motivated than those of
Falloppio. One seeming exception is a passage in which Rudio tells of
a recent case in his experience: an infected mother, after a stillbirth,
nursed two orphaned infants; they were almost immediately infected
and died a painful death. Rudio concludes: "But she will find that
God avenges such a disgraceful action and crime."[30] But perhaps
rather than a deep religious conviction this sentence shows an understandable human or even humanist outrage, fed also by a sense of the
physician's utter helplessness.

Rudio presents one of the few suggestions about how women
can avoid becoming infected (a pessary steeped in a concoction of
"Indian wood" [guaiac] is to be worn a whole day after intercourse),
but even so, his perspective is so secular-humanistic-male as to strike
us as inhumane: Rudio speaks of "paid women, who are worth preserving not for their own health, but primarily for the sake of their
male customers."[31] Just as Falloppio's words were directed to his students less as future diagnosticians, counselors, and healers than as
users of that medical knowledge in their personal lives, so Rudio's are
addressed to single men (among whom he seems to include himself
[p. 168]), whom he admonishes to exercise caution should a woman
offer herself to them. This caution, however, is not equivalent to absolute abstinence. Rudio tells the case of a young man who inserted his
member only, as he swore by oath, "for a single moment" (*soli quasi
momento temporis*, p. 169), until he felt some hardness in the woman's
pudenda that made him suspect that she had the French disease. Nevertheless this man caught the infection and soon was ravaged by the
disease. Rudio wants to have this matter (so graphically) expressed
"for the common good" or "common health" (*pro communi saluti*, [p.
169]), and recommends that his students retract immediately and
interrupt the act when noticing suspicious symptoms in the woman's
genital area.

If "common health" (*salus communis*) appears to be focused on
the health of men, there are passages—and they are among Rudio's
most forceful ones—where he has in mind even more narrowly the

health of physicians. Since he considers a doctor's infection with the *virus Gallicum* a public shame, these passages relate to the topic of medical ethics as a more limited topic of physicians' professional ethics as perceived by the public. Thus his concern is not, as one might expect from the modern perspective, to warn physicians of the danger of contracting the disease while treating a diseased patient, but to impress on them the need to be cautious in their sexual habits. In his estimation, a good thousand men in medicine have been infected by women whom they thought true and faithful Penelopes (p. 168). And he adds: "This warning here I have meant to issue for the physicians' health. For if it is shameful that others are deceived, it will be most shameful if those who profess the art of medicine are made to shipwreck."[32] He describes the dilemma of two doctors known to him years before who were graced by the most beautiful beards. After losing those beards through the effects of syphilis, both had to leave Venice to avoid public ridicule and shame (pp. 168–69).

In his extraordinarily graphic and concrete passages about prevention, whether talking about loss of hair, coitus interruptus, or forms of lascivious kisses that transmit the virus (p. 169), Rudio indicates awareness of stretching accepted bounds of decorum. His justification is the appeal to a *salus communis* and *salus medicorum*, concepts which, although not strictly defined and somewhat overlapping, are with him essentially secular.

Daniel Sennert's Response to Falloppio

The reaction of Falloppio's contemporary, Protestant Henri Estienne (see the previous section), prepares us for the response of the widely acclaimed Daniel Sennert (1572–1637), Professor at Wittenberg in the early seventeenth century. What could be discussed at Padua in the middle of the sixteenth century apparently was not sayable in Protestant Wittenberg several decades later.

In the chapter, "On Prevention," of his treatise on venereal disease, Daniel Sennert sharply criticizes Falloppio and the tradition of writing on prevention deriving from him, although, as we shall see, Sennert's view is somewhat contradictory. According to the English translation of 1660, he says:

Wheneas 'tis safer to prevent a Disease than to cure it, some Physitians endeavor to teach, by what means one may keep himself clear, though he have had to do with an infected Woman. Of which business *Falloppio* treats in the whol Chapter, 89 *De Morb. Galli*, and he writes that he should seem to have done nothing unless he teach, how one seeing a handsome Woman, and lying with her though infected, may be preserved from the French Disease: and he calls the immortal God to witness, that he hath made tryal of it in ten thousand (*sic*) men, and none of them was infected: and he propounds there two medicaments, by which the Contagion received may presently be drawn forth, dissipated, or dryed up."[33]

By calling attention to the appeal to "the immortal God to witness," Sennert teases out the contradiction between Falloppio's seeming encouragement to sin even more boldly (fortified by the preventive measures) and the Italian's somewhat conventional or even routine religiosity that allows Falloppio to call upon God to guarantee the veracity of his discourse. He charges that syphilographers in the tradition of Falloppio (including Ercole Sassonia and Eustachio Rudio) give people a sense of security so that, guarded with these medicines "as with a buckler" (*tamquam clypeo*), they "enter the most infected Whores, and freely ramble all the world over" (p. 27). Sennert thus seems to disagree with the principle of such prevention: "But indeed I do not believe, that those things can be taught with a good conscience, by which so many men are encouraged to lust, whom perhaps the fear of this disease might have frightened from it; and therefore we will say nothing of these medicines."[34] Sennert indeed does not report Falloppio's preventive stratagems, most notably the *linteolum* (small linen cloth) cut and shaped to the size of the penis and steeped in certain lotions, and if he had ended his chapter on prevention with this morally charged figure of omission (*praeteritio*), one would have to grant his stance a logical and moral consistency. But Sennert does not stop here.

Drawing on Aurelio Minadoi (fl. 1596),[35] Sennert now wonders whether Falloppio and the others following him are not deceived about the nature of the infection: perhaps the disease is not communicated only "by very small purulent corpuscles" (*per minima corpuscula saniosa*) which can be wiped away. "He [Minadoi] teacheth that the Contagion does not only enter by the external parts of the Privities, but also chiefly by the internal, and runs through the Body, and that the infected Vapors, and spirits do pass through the internal porosities, and are admitted by the Veins" (p. 27). With hardly a touch of the moral indignation that informs Sennert's reaction to Falloppio, Minadoi had argued that the "shield" was only imaginary, and in addition to the internal porosities of the genitals, there was also oral infection.[36] For Sennert, the consequence of this doubt about the kind of prevention advocated by Falloppio is clear: "Therefore no man can promise himself health and safetie from washing, which only reaches to the external parts, nor from other Medicaments outwardly applied, neither can such external Medicaments take away the Pollution conceived within. The safest way therefore to avoid this disease is to abstain from whores, and to remember that Whoremongers and Adulterers the Lord will judge, who is wont also to punish them in this Life, with the most filthy Disease" (pp. 27–28). Even this view has some limited consistency: one should not teach prevention that induces people to sin more boldly. The moral-theological view is supplemented (if not supported) by the medical consideration that the sense of safety from the disease may be false. This means of prevention may not be effective—two good reasons, then, why Sennert does not mention Falloppio's *linteolum*.

But Sennert does not leave matters at that, going on to report that the physician Palmarius (Julien Le Paulmier de Grentemesnil [1520–1588], disciple of the celebrated Jean Fernel) has another means of preventing this disease, namely an internal medication. This antidote or "mullet" is claimed to make the body impervious to the infection:

> Yet he [Palmarius] entreats and conjures al Physitians and Chyrurgeons, that they do not communicate and make known that Medicine in obedience to lustful people, and that they make not themselves fosterers of lusts, but to them only who must necessarily converse with those that are suspected or defiled. But he describes that Antidote, Lib. 1 cap. 8. and this is it. (p. 28)

Then follows the recipe and dosage, printed for everyone to see.

To some extent Sennert is here reproducing the inconsistencies of the French physician's moral stance in his chapter, "Precaution Against Lues Venerea." Palmarius had said that "if someone intends to avoid *lues venerea*, he will either have to abstain entirely from illicit coition (*impurus concubitus*) and other venereal contact, which Christians ought to do anyway, or else so prepare and arm his body that it will admit least of it."[37] After referring to the proverbial King Mithridates as his model (who by frequently imbibing an alexipharmacum is supposed to have made his body eventually resistant to poison), Palmarius had indeed claimed to have "found" or "invented" (*invenimus*) such an antidote against venereal disease. Since he did not want base whoremongers go free of the dire punishment for their shameful acts (*gravissimae flagitiorum suorum poena*) but rather have them rein in their lusts by considering God's wrath and vengeance (*numinis ira et ultio*), Palmarius had indeed, as Sennert reports, implored physicians and surgeons to keep his "amulet" from the wrong people. But finally Sennert's account takes another turn: after printing the recipe for the French physician's amulet or antidote, Sennert adds the skeptical note: "But whenas all those simple Medicaments, which are in the Antidote, are not proper to this Venereal Disease, we must consult with experience, whether their virtue be so great, as *Palmarius* cries it up for."

Sennert's chapter on the prevention of venereal disease is unusually challenging. I consulted the Latin text hoping to find that some of the difficulties were the result of a moralizing English translator. But the translation is quite accurate: the bobbing and weaving is all Sennert's. At least three explanations of this tortuous movement of the text can be offered. It might be said that some of the contradictions are the result of the principle of inclusiveness or completeness, so powerful in the prescientific era, a principle that impelled a Robert Burton to collect everything available on the subject of melancholy, even if he was unable (in spite of repeated attempts to divide and order) to shape the contradictory elements into an entirely coherent new whole. Second, Sennert's moral sense, which dictated both his attack on Falloppio and his withholding of the Italian's preventive measures, may have been a little shallow, since after the broadside on Falloppio Sennert did not hesitate to give the details of Palmarius's internal "antidote," in possible violation of the Frenchman's insistent request not to divulge it to potential abusers. Finally, Sennert's way of revealing some measures of prevention and concealing others might still have been controlled by the same moral sensibility: in spite of Minadoi's reported skepticism, Sennert might have feared that readers could be seduced by the authority of Falloppio to rely on his preventive prescriptions and engage in sex acts both illicit and injurious to their health. Minadoi, on the other hand, was pretty much a medical unknown, the *tractatus* being his only publication.[38] There is even the possibility that Sennert, although registering Minadoi's skepticism, might himself have been attracted to the view that the prevention advocated by Falloppio would work. As to Palmarius, who, as Jean Fernel's student, was better known than Minadoi but certainly not of the eminence of Falloppio, Sennert might have considered his own reservations about the Frenchman's antidote, the simples of which were not specifically indicated for the new disease, persuasive enough to discourage reliance upon it; but since commission on Sennert's part is at least as bothersome as omission, this latter point must remain hypothetical.

Sennert's ideas on venereal disease are important partly because, translated into English, they had considerable impact on an English public familiar only with the vernacular. At the end of the century, the anonymous author of "Some Curious Problems," in *A Method of Curing the French-Pox* (London, 1690), allegedly a Frenchman, follows the tortuous movement of Sennert's argument surprisingly closely when writing his Problem VII, entitled, "If there be any infallible Preservative against the Venereal Distemper." These are the opening sentences of a detailed answer:

> Libertines have been, for a long time, searching for some preventing Medicine to Arm them against the Venereal Distemper, that they might continue their dissolute Life, and yet be without the reach of that Disease. We also see, that some Authors do give Prescriptions for this purpose; from which some promise themselves marvellous Success, and are very confident, that by that means, Men may take their swing, keep as much company as they do please with Persons infected with the Venereal Distemper. By this, all Men of Sence may easily judge, that such Authors are Cheats, which to purchase Credit at the cost of others, do venture all at one, and so prostitute their Conscience, which must needs be struck with horror, for teaching a Remedy in favour of a debauched Conversation. . . . (p. 117)

With such a "remedy," the anonymous author argues, males would flock to the "stews," just as young women (according to the anonymous author) would not value virginity if they had a contraceptive. Then he takes the same turn as Sennert, "All such Preservatives, to speak properly, are nothing else but Impostures" (p. 118), possibly achieving a little more precision by adding: "the most conclusive is

such, as at most, does only prove the possibility of such a Remedy."
Like Sennert, the anonymous author then launches into a discussion
of "talismans" as he remembers "men who being fortified with good
Antidotes did so vigorously defend themselves against Poyson that
they suffered no alteration from them"—a version of Palmarius's reference to Mithridates. He gives credence to such talismans for preventing the plague, but apparently not venereal disease; the reason is
that God sees no need for it:

> But, as to the Venereal Distemper, seeing that it is commonly the
> reward of the Sin of Fornication, which God has always had in
> Abomination, and that that Distemper may be avoided by Conti-
> nence, which is the true Preservative, it seems that it was no
> ways necessary that God should create a specific Preservative
> against that. (p. 120)

Although largely paralleling Sennert's argument, the anonymous author goes beyond him in one respect, namely in raising the
question of the plight of those guiltlessly infected by the disease:

> And for those, being innocent, have contracted the Venereal Dis-
> temper, as Infants in the Mother's Womb, or on the Breasts, Vir-
> tuous Women who have got it from their dissolute Husbands,
> and those good Husbands that are trespass'd by their extrava-
> gant Wives; It is sufficient, that there are assured Medicines in
> Nature, and in the hands of skilful Artists for the Cure of that
> Distemper. (p. 120)

Here ethical curiosity is apparently quickly stinted by moral-religious
justification, a seemingly easy theodicy that minimizes human suffering. The author does not go far beyond Sennert.

Sennert fits into the intellectual landscape of Europe somewhere
between, on the one hand, the Italian syphilographers willing to fur-
nish their students with the prophylaxis that would allow them to
enjoy compliant women safely and yet capable of invoking God for a
witness in the same context and, on the other, the English surgeons
and physicians writing on the subject, imbued with values that make
them view almost every aspect of the disease through a moral lens.
(That the English works are in the vernacular and might have been
considered more easily misused by their authors may skew the

comparison slightly, but not significantly. Clearly Falloppio's lectures, although in Latin, attracted a varied, though of course entirely male, audience.) Between the physicians in Italy, whose interest in preventing disease is so immediate and seemingly without reflection that they feel no need to justify it, and the Englishmen, whose moral stance is consistent with their silence on prevention (but whose medical stance may have its contradictions), the Wittenberg professor articulates his moral opposition to a prevention that he believes will make men morally irresponsible. But at the same time genuine doubts were being raised about the effectiveness of Falloppio's ideas or about any kind of prevention, doubts Sennert thought it his duty to communicate. If these doubts were justified, the entire matter seemed to shift back from being a moral problem to a primarily medical one. Perhaps because the unsettled question of medical effectiveness then could be seen as superseding the moral question of prevention or as taking priority over it, Sennert was unable to address with greater clarity the possible conflicts between a physician's medical and moral duties. Obviously such Renaissance discussions relate to pressing issues of our day, for instance to what has been called "the clash of pragmatism and morality."[39]

Ultimately, Sennert may also have lacked the tools that had been sharpened by the *canonistae* and *summistae* in a long tradition of moral casuistry, terms like "commission" and "omission," as well as various categories of conditional speech and indirect enticement. Another limitation, which he shared with most physicians of his time, was that he perceived the dangers of venereal disease primarily in terms of dangers to men. Tapping into the large reservoir of Roman Catholic casuist thinking and using the important ethicist and physician Paolo Zacchia (1584–1659) as an intermediary, Giovanni Battista Sitoni, an Italian physician of a curiously "feminist" temper, was soon to challenge the Italian secular teaching about syphilis (for which he chose Sassonia as his prime and negative example) as misguided in order to advocate a medical ethics guided by higher norms.

Women and the Origin of Syphilis

In the previous section we traced Renaissance ideas according to which particular groups of people or individual nations are punished with syphilis, as well as the ways such moralized views of pathology inform Renaissance ideas about prevention. For us these ideas adum-

brate the modern dilemma of ethicists whether to recommend abstinence or use of condoms.[40] Anna Foa has shown how, during the first
few decades after the appearance of syphilis in central Europe, the
tendency was to make an "other" responsible for it: it was the disease
of the French, Italian, American Indian, or the Jew.[41] However,
beyond incidental comments (for instance, by Foa and Anthony
Grafton), no one has yet studied in detail how women figure in these
early speculations about the origin and transmission of a deadly disease. This is surprising since early ideas about syphilis offer a more
powerful argument for the social construction of disease and its
nexus with gender than complex recent examples like chlorosis and
AIDS, through which that argument has been proposed. Further, as
we will see, one rather special (and admittedly rare) application of
the gendered form of these ideas in the Renaissance was to elicit in
the mid-seventeenth century a wide-ranging attack on a secular medical ethics.[42] In fact, one cannot read far into the works of Renaissance
syphilographers without being struck by the gendered perceptions of
syphilis in the period.

Pervasive in so many contexts of Renaissance physicians' writing about this disease is the assumption that women are the agents,
the active infectors. Philip Barrough's comment on the dangers of the
French disease may stand for the most general form of this assumption: "There be develish women desirous to be handled and dealt
withall, who will beautifie themselves, to inflame mens hearts to lust
towards them."[43] Ercole Sassonia (1551–1607), in the period celebrated as a distinguished medical practitioner and author, believed
that at least sometimes the disease is caused by excessive heat of the
vulva.[44] Occasionally the view was held that syphilis arose from sexual intercourse during menstruation. The modern reader may immediately recognize this hypothesis as another way to hold women
responsible. However, an anonymous (allegedly French) medical
author (whom I quote in a translation of the seventeenth century)
interprets this as a fabrication to *excuse* women:

> There is frequently a specious Pretext used to palliate the the
> Crimes of such Women as have given the Venereal Distemper to
> their Husbands, by telling them, that the mischief has therefore
> befallen them, because they would needs embrace them whilst
> they had their Courses. There are some who tell some Old Wom-
> en's Stories, or some Passages taken out of *Cardan, John Baptista*

Porta, or the Book of *Albertus Magnus, de secretis mulierum.* They alledge that the Vapour of the *Menstrua* does stain Looking-glasses, so as no man can remove the Infection, that Women kill the Plants that are near them....[45]

This explanation of the origin of syphilis, here effectively ridiculed, obviously makes use of the view of the menses as poisonous, a view strongly opposed by the well-known physician Mercuriale (1530–1606, who was held in high esteem by Pope Pius IV and Emperor Maximilian II). But Mercuriale's view gained acceptance only gradually over what is here, in a gendered polemic, called "Old Women's Stories." (If, as late as the eighteenth century, the notoriously commercial publisher Curll could market an English translation of the *de secretis* enticingly as on the secrets of women, it may not be surprising to find the notion of the poisonous menstrual discharge very much alive in the seventeenth.)[46]

Pietro Rostino (sixteenth century), who wrote a popular tract on syphilis (in Italian), thought that all infectious diseases were caused by some form of humidity (that swamps are unhealthy is a medical commonplace, reappearing in different guise also in Fracastoro's notion of infectious *seminaria* arising from humid places). In the case of syphilis, the "humidity" (according to Rostino) was supplied by the ulcerated pudenda of a woman during intercourse. According to another hypothesis about the origin of the French disease, neither the menses nor ulcers in the woman's organs but leprous infections were the catalyst. According to Gaspar Torrella (1452–1520), the disease erupted after a leprous knight on the way to the Italian campaign had intercourse with a woman at Valencia, who then infected many other men.[47] A little later, Thierry de Héry (ca. 1500–1560), who accompanied Francis I in 1539 on his ill-fated Italian campaign (during which Héry learned to treat the disease that, as he boasted, was to make his fortune), has a more precise version of what seems to be the same encounter: "The authors say, and it is the most common opinion, that when King Charles VIII went to Italy in 1493 to put down Naples, a leprous knight at Valencia in Spain bought a night with a woman for 50 ecus, who afterward infected several young men sleeping with her, several of whom followed the king's train."[48]

I am reporting this hypothesis in detail because it is close to the theory of origin that Paracelsus (1493–1541) is alleged to have had. In his *Chirurgia magna* (1536), he said that syphilis came from the intercourse of a leprous Frenchman and a prostitute with uterine sores,[49] and it seems to be this passage that, in the seventeenth century, Stephen Blankaart has in mind when he reports without giving his source that Paracelsus attributed the outbreak of the French disease to a leprous prostitute in 1478.[50] However, either Paracelsus was vacillating between different explanatory attempts or he arrived at the one just named only gradually; for the Latin and German versions of Paracelsus's *Vom Ursprung und Herkommen der Franzosen* (1529) are slightly different. Here, at the beginning of bk. 1, chap. 1, Paracelsus indeed gives a pre-Columbian date for the outbreak of the disease (1480) and (without reference to a prostitute) attributes it to *luxuria* (voluptuousness) at the moment of conception. In the following chapters, particularly chapter 5, he stresses the proximity of the disease to leprosy.[51] For a compiler like Blankaart, Paracelsus's view was important, although Paracelsus seems to have borrowed the attribution of the origin of the disease to leprous women from other physicians. Indeed, in the first half of the sixteenth century, Pietro Andrea Mattioli, personal physician to two emperors, says he has this version from "several" informants or authors (*nonnulli*).[52]

Finally, and perhaps most interestingly in my context, there is a theory which, for convenience, I will quote from *A New Method of Curing the French-Pox*, since it is in English. The already adduced anonymous (and allegedly French) author of that book subscribes to it. (An earlier version can be found in Giovanni Tommaso Minadoi, another highly reputed physician and professor at Padua, who died in 1615.)

> But 'tis known, that if a Virgin, that is perfectly sound (if the Matter be so ordered as to free her from all suspicion of the Venereal Distemper) shall keep Company with half a dozen young Fellows, as sound as herself, and be debauched with them severally, time after time, some one or other of them shall quickly have the Pox, and all of them, by a repetition of Venereal Acts, shall at last be infected. (p. 3)

The French disease is thus imagined to arise without extraneous infection, a scenario that would most commonly hold in the case of prostitutes. Our author restates the matter, perhaps slightly more ambiguously, but adding what to him is the crucial element of the theory:

I suppose that a common Woman has the Pox, and though she were not infected, if she has a particular Conversation [intercourse] with many Men, the mixture of so many Seeds does occasion such a Corruption in the Passage of the Matrix, that it degenerates into a proper virulent Ferment. . . . (p. 20)

The author explains at length and by various analogies how he imagines the "venereal ferment" to develop into the "venereal distemper": still holding, according to the Galenic tradition, that women also have seeds, he thinks that "the Seeds of one Man and of one Woman only can never degenerate into contagion and Venereal Ferment . . ." (p. 29). This leads him to the conclusion that "it shall therefore happen when a Common Woman has kept company with many Men, that the Seeds (which are of different, and often times of opposite qualities) being mixed into that womans Womb (which is naturally fitted to preserve the Seeds and all their Spirits) do forcibly justle against one another" (pp. 29–30), and the resulting agitation leads to the ferment, which turns into the venereal distemper.

In this scenario (clearly shown also in the hypothetical case of the virgin turning promiscuous), the woman's body becomes the locus of corruption (for which she would also be primarily responsible) and the vehicle of the infection of others. At the risk of overinterpretation, I venture to add that the notion of spirits of male seed in conflict (unnaturally locked in as it were) leading to the corruption of syphilis also has a homophobic element, a version possibly of the homophobic shudder that can be observed elsewhere in the period.[53]

Syphilis and the Power of Virgins

In his well-known *Instruction of a Christian Woman*, which was translated into many vernacular languages, the famous humanist Juan Luis Vives (1492–1540) reports the following case of a married couple at Bruges. I am quoting the most important parts (of what Vives presents as an eyewitness account) from a Renaissance translation, but supplying some words from the Latin original:

Clare the wyfe of Barnarde Valdaure, a fayre and goodly mayde (*virgo tenerrima et formosissima*), whan she was fyrste maryed at Bruges, and brought to bedde unto her husband, whiche was 46

yere of age (*iam plus quadraginta annos natum*), the fyrste nyghte
saw his legges rolled and wrapped with cloutes (*crura eius fasciis
involuta vidit*), and founde that she had chaunced on a sore and
sickely husband: yet for all that, she lothed hym never the more,
nor beganne nat to hate hym: whom yet she had no space to
love (*quum praesertim nondum posset videri amare*). Not long after
that, the forsayde Valdaure fell into a great syckeness, in so
moche that all the phisitions dispayred his lyfe: than she and her
mother gave such dilygence unto the sicke man, that for syx
wekes continually together, neyther of them ones put of their
clothes, excepte it were to chaunge the smockes: nor rested in
the nyghte paste one houre, or iii at the most, and that but in
their clothes. The roote of the disease was, that we call the
french pockes, (*erat radix morbi Indici, quem Gallicum hic vocant*),
a wonderous sore and contagious sickness, phisitions counsayled her, nat to touche him so, nor come so nere hym: and the
same, her friendes counsayled her. And her companions and
gossyppes said: it was synfully done, to vexe the man in the
worlde, or kepe him longer on live with his sickenes, and bad
her provide some good thynge for the soule, as for the bodye
care no more, but howe it myght be buryed. . . . Soo at the laste
by the goode meanes of his wyfe, Valdaure escaped the great
ieoperdye, that both the phisitions, and all other men swered,
his wyfe had plucked hym from deth by stronge hande. And
some iested more merily than becommeth christen folkes, and
sayd, that god had purposed to have slaine Valdaure, but his
wyfe wolde not let him go out of her handes. . . . Streight after
he fell in to an other longe disease, which lasted vii yere. . . .
Moreover whan the ayre of hym and breth was such, that no
man myght abyde nere by ten passes, she wolde swere, that she
thought it marveylous swe[e]te: And once she was very angrye
with me, bycause I sayd it stanke, for she sayd, it semed unto
here lyke the savour of rype and swete frute. . . . So he by the
meanes of his wyfe, with that dolefull body, more lyke unto a
grave than a body (*cadaveroso corpore, seu sepulchro verius*), continued ten yere from the begynning of his sycknes, in the whiche
space she had two chyldren by hym, and six before. For she was
married xx yere in the holle: and yet was never infected, nor
ones touched with the contagious scabbe, neither she nor yet
none of her chyldren, but had all their bodyes both holle and

clene. Wherby a man may clerely perceyve, how moch theyr holynes and virtue is worthe (*ex quo liquidum sit quanta sit virtus*), that love their housbandes with all theyr hartes as dutie is, whiche doubtless god wyll never leave unrewarded.[54]

While the passages attributing agency in the genesis of the disease to women (discussed in the previous section) are perhaps revealing to modern intellectual historians, there is one topic centrally located in the field of medical ethics that called for conscious reflection on gender roles as early as the seventeenth century: the notion that sexual intercourse with a virgin could cure an infected male of syphilis. To counter the objection that fortunately even then the idea may have belonged more to the area of folklore and superstition than to medicine, I have quoted Vives's case of Clara Cerventa and Bernard Valdaura, who were in fact Vives's parents-in-law. Obviously the case fits my context only imperfectly: Vives tells it in his chapter entitled, "Quomodo se erga maritum habebit" (how she will conduct herself toward her husband), and there is no suggestion that the *virgo tenerrima* cured her husband instantly by sleeping with him—after all, he had what we would call "relapses," and died (twenty years later) apparently of the same disease. But "she plucked hym from deth" to the astonishment of the community, and in the largest Renaissance compendium of received knowledge, the *Theatrum vitae humanae*, by the Swiss physician Theodor Zwinger (1533–1588), the story is summarized as a cure from syphilis by a virgin.[55] Although Vives's modern biographer finds its realism "revolting,"[56] the case is so redolent of sixteenth-century life that one may be allowed to ask a question that Vives most pointedly does *not* ask, namely what Bernard Valdaura's motives for marriage were: did he merely want a nurse or did he hope to be healed from his disease by the *virtus* of the *virgo tenerrima*? As in the previous chapter on the treatment of hysteria, we are dealing with a subject that is of course highly tabooed, although the proof texts demonstrating the special sensitivity that the topic elicited are in this case even later. But since in the seventeenth century earlier authors are castigated for ever mentioning the belief that virgins might heal syphilitics, it is possible that the outrage Erasmus articulated against pairing diseased men with healthy young women in his colloquy *Coniugium impar* (Unequal Marriage), and even Alciati's emblem "Nupta contagiosa" (comparing such a marriage to being chained to a corpse), may have this belief as an unmentionable background.[57]

The notion that virgins have the power to heal syphilis has left some interesting echoes in the works of at least two physicians. In his *Luis venereae perfectissimus tractatus* (1597), Hercole Sassonia raises the following problem in a chapter entitled "De gonorrhaea antiqua":

> But one needs to inquire into what I have heard was experienced by some people in Venice: they claim [*dicunt*] to have been cured instantly of gonorrhea by having intercourse with a Black woman [*mulier Aethiopis*]. The *experimentum* [experience; experiment; demonstration or proof] is true and it seems can be confirmed by [Julius Caesar] Scaliger's *exercitatio* 180, c. 18, according to whom Africans are cured from lues venerea by sleeping with a Numidian or Ethiopian woman. That I know, too, even though I would consider as invented the reports that indeed more men were freed from *gonorrhaea antiqua* by sleeping with a virgin spouse; but then the woman gets infected.[58]

In his *Exoticarum exercitationum liber*, Julius Caesar Scaliger (1484–1553) indeed reports that in Africa (where, according to him, the disease was first imported by Jewish refugees expelled from Spain), "those suffering from it recover, by a gift merely of the Heavens, by sleeping with a Numidian or Black Ethiopian woman, without any other medications."[59] Perhaps Sassonia felt some uneasiness about the moral interpretation of this remedy as a "gift of the Heavens," or else his secular temperament makes him drop or reduce such interpretation generally. But he did not express his uneasiness clearly. His inaccuracy about section and chapter numbers in Scaliger is minor. But there are more serious problems with Sassonia's passage.

First, an ambiguity about what Sassonia reports to be "true" (*verum*) is somewhat troubling: "they say" (*dicunt*) they have been cured in this special way—is it true that they say so (i.e. is it true that people making such claims exist?), or is it the content of their claim true? Most troubling is the form *consignam*: is it a printer's misreading of *consignari*? (As we shall see, a seventeenth-century reader and fluent Latinist did not think so.) Then there is the possibility that *consignare literis* should not be translated idiomatically as "record," but as "to assign to letters," i.e. a realm differing somehow in status from reality. Finally, a punctuation mark may be missing after *consignam*, resulting in ambiguity as to what Sassonia wants to "note," "record," or "assign to letters": what precedes the verb (the

Numidian and Ethiopian story) or what follows (namely the general cure by virgins). By choosing the latter reading, my translation may be said to give Sassonia the benefit of the doubt and avoid the more obnoxious reading. If however, a syntactic break after *consignam* was intended (which could have been, but need not have been, indicated by a mark of punctuation), Sassonia is saying that several or "more" (*plures*) have been cured in this way. If we accept the Latin as it is, nothing is ambiguous about the final sentence: Sassonia knows for certain, as the verb in the indicative indicates, that the woman gets infected in this process. As we shall see, not everyone gave Sassonia the benefit of the doubt.

Sassonia was taken to task in the seventeenth century by the physician Giovanni Battista Sitoni (1605–1681), who discussed the matter under the chapter heading: "Whether a man suffering from the French disease will be cured of the disease by intercourse with a virgin?"[60] To my knowledge, Sitoni is the first physician to emphasize that man and woman both labor under the scourge of venereal disease. In fact, the discussion of this farsighted Milanese physician (on whom the standard biographical dictionary by August Hirsch is disappointingly brief) has a preface that we may call (admittedly anachronistically) "feminist" on the relative value of man and woman. It concludes that both are "correlative" (*correlativa*, p. 288). Far from being a commonplace at that time, the idea of their correlative nature becomes a focal point of Sitoni's argument.

Sitoni is possibly also the first to say with similar emphasis that the disease "is not only transmitted from women to men but (since it is reciprocal) also from men to women."[61] In this context Sitoni reports that "nevertheless a certain remedy of this scourge is pranked up as if it could serve as the safest cure of infected men," namely coition with a virgin.[62] Sitoni objects that there is no truth to the claim, nor can there be, for it would be just as absurd to claim that an infected woman could be cured of the disease by sleeping with an inexperienced male. He is so fond of this argument, derived from his axiom of the correlative nature of man and woman, that he will repeat it later in even greater detail (p. 292). He assigns the presumed powers of virginity to mere popular belief (*credit vulgus*, p. 291) and, drawing on humoral physiology, reasons that coition does not change the balance of the patient's humors, which (according to Galen) would be necessary for a cure. In any case, he reports, experience tells us only that when syphilitic men marry virgins, they infect them without in the least being cured of the disease: he has not seen a single case where such a man was healed.

All this is preparation for taking on the famous physician and syphilographer Ercole Sassonia. "In this respect we say that the presentation of the most learned Sassonia . . . is insufficient when he writes the following." As he then quotes, Sitoni does not give Sassonia the benefit of the doubt. In fact, he inserts a colon in the critical space after the verb *consignam* (which he amends to *consignem*), making sure that Sassonia is not read as assigning to letters (fiction?) the cure of *plures* by their virgin spouses, but that his skepticism refers to what precedes the verb. (He also changes *licet* to *scilicet*.) Thus he has Sassonia say: "That [i.e. the habits of Africans] I know, too, even though I would consider it letters [fiction?]; more men were evidently freed from *gonorrhaea antiqua* by sleeping with a virgin spouse, but then the woman is being infected."[63] Possibly because he reads the sentence as casting some doubt on the African practices, Sitoni does not separately raise the issue whether Sassonia's passage might induce someone to look for a Black woman. Sitoni charges that the counsel he interprets Sassonia to be proffering is governed by the subtlety of lust rather than the desire for health; it behooves no decent man to deceive some poor young virgin and, by the ruse of seeking health, expose her to such a scourge, putting her life at the highest risk. He adds that "a believing physician" (*pius medicus*) should not offer such advice to anyone, since he would be advocating something "novel and voluptuous," i.e. would be going beyond accepted modes of cure.

He reasons in even more detail that such medical advice would either lead to "illicit" intercourse (with just any virgin) or to a "licit" act (with a virgin married just for that purpose). Advice to do the former is improper, since it is an accepted principle of ethics that one should neither commit, nor advise anyone to commit, any act in the interest of health that leads to sin. Here he refers among others to Zacchia (1584–1659), protomedicus of the Vatican and personal physician of Innocent X and Alexander VII, and to the physician Codronchi (sixteenth century), author of the often quoted book on Christian (and decidedly Catholic) medical ethics that I have adduced several times (particularly in chapter 4). Advice to do the latter, i.e. to marry a virgin for the sake of health, is improper for the same reason, and Sitoni lists a number of legal and medical authorities (among the latter Rodrigo a Castro) for the traditional principle to stick with "safe and certain" (*tuta et certa*) remedies. He points out that it is an equally accepted principle not to ruin the welfare of one for the sake of that of another and makes explicit what was perhaps not always implied, namely that the life of a woman is to be valued as much as that of a man (p. 294). Since offspring are traditionally the major purpose of licit intercourse (while with the wife's infection no healthy offspring, if any at all, can be expected), medical counsel to enter matrimony for such an extraneous reason would endanger the patient's spiritual health in this respect also. That such action is neither to be committed nor to be counseled "not only all Canonists conclude, but also all physicians thinking as Catholics."[64]

The phrase *medici catholice sentientes* is typical of Zacchia's grouping of medical authorities and is indeed used by the canonist/physician Zacchia in a very similar context (without, however, referring to this presumed remedy for syphilis).[65] Since all Sitoni's references on this problem of extraneous reasons for marriage are also in Zacchia and precisely so (except that Sitoni erroneously drops a digit in a reference to a chapter by Codronchi—it should be 20, as Zacchia has it), Sitoni was undoubtedly following Zacchia, perhaps exclusively.

Given the scarcity of my information about Sitoni, I can only offer surmises as to why he so deftly took to task the earlier physician, who enjoyed a high reputation and is almost universally referred to with utmost respect. Particularly his strong feeling about gender equity, which I loosely called "feminist," must unfortunately remain inexplicable. But beyond that, it is clear that his sensibility is formed by writers like Zacchia and the *canonistae* behind him. On the very page of Zacchia that Sitoni must have consulted on the subject of the inadmissibility of medical counsel endangering the patient's soul (and from which he took the phrase *medici catholice sentientes*), Sitoni would have found Zacchia adducing the canonists for their opposition also to indirect, conditional, or ambiguous counsel that could induce the patient to sin. Specifically Zacchia quoted the Roman Catholic moral casuist Navarra's example: "I do not advise you to do so, but if you do this or this, you will recover," and agreed with the Spaniard that such conditional speech was inadmissible. Sitoni would have found Zacchia deliberately going even one step further in also ruling out speech "by exception," of which he gave this example: "If its sinfullness did not argue against it, intercourse would restore your health."[66] Unquestionably Sitoni's suspicion that Sassonia was engaging in such forms of indirect counsel triggered his outrage. However dubious his way of repunctuating the earlier physician's sentence may be by modern standards of scholarship, his "revision," or editing, was only explicating one particular way in which Sassonia's ambiguous sentence could in fact be read; and ambiguity, like indirectness, could lead to results that were obnoxious.

But was Sitoni not using the very mode Zacchia chastised in his example, namely saying that such intercourse for the purpose of recovery from disease was sinful yet thereby indirectly encouraging or at least tempting some desperate males to consider this action? Of course not. He unambiguously said that cure from syphilis could not be gained by intercourse—while Sassonia had been ambiguous, an ambiguity that could lead to irreparable harm.

I am less certain about a related matter, the occasion of the essay. This particular piece (tractatus 45) of his *Miscellanea medico-curiosa* is dedicated to Count (*comes*) Iacobo Francisco Attendolo, who is addressed personally at the end. The author expresses his hope that the addressee, convalescing from a sudden fever, will not loathe perusing the essay, for "so the opportunity of the hour urges, which provides festivities (*bacchanalia*) to those whom the calamity of the present war does not cause to mourn."[67] Most likely these are polite sentences of "paratextual" wrapping, quite conventional in this genre, referring to a contemporary occasion unimportant for the subject of the piece. But there is at least the possibility that the somewhat elliptic language is coded, namely that the "fever" from which the *comes illustrissimus* is suffering is a euphemism, and that he personally could profit from the argument.

Ercole Sassonia (whose moral sense is critiqued by Sitoni) is one of the most secular-minded writers on syphilis we have reviewed, and it may not be surprising that he struck a seventeenth-century reader as objectionable. Thus, on the subject of *lues venerea* in conjunction with fever, Sassonia reports two successful cures from that fever: one was Petrus Basalù, "still living and healthy"; the other was Nicoleta, "a most well-known prostitute in Venice, who after suffering for four continuous years from *Hectica Venerea* and through that period always being confined to her bed, was restored to health through a concoction of Indian wood, so that she can at this time again practice the meretricious art."[68] Unlike Rudio, whose revealing comment we noted earlier, Sassonia does not feel impelled to explain or excuse his treating prostitutes. That Nicoleta returned to practicing the "art" is part of his story of her successful cure, a matter of professional pride, and not cause for moral reflection.

Thus this vignette of the cure of a prostitute can serve as an example of medical praxis illustrating the more secular frame of mind one finds in some Italian writers on syphilis but also, more generally, in such an articulate writer on both medical ethics and women's diseases as Rodrigo a Castro. In his work on medical ethics, Castro had criticized physicians who, out of excessive zeal (*ex nimio zelo*), chide or castigate their patients for their vices rather than putting them at ease.[69] We saw earlier (in chapter 3) that when Castro, an expatriate from Portugal, was attacked for being Jewish by malevolent and self-serving detractors, his apologists defended him, saying, "Physicians do not concern themselves with conscience, with the health of the soul, but with the health of the body and the remedy and cure of diseases."[70] This view, a polemical sharpening of secular trends in Galenic medicine, was precisely the position in medical ethics that Sitoni resented and which he wanted to challenge by writing his piece. Unfortunately Sitoni does not identify the *quisquam* (someone) whose view he cites and ridicules by applying it to the case in point (the "cure" of sleeping with a virgin):

> The physician who is a sensitive [*sensitivus* = "feeling"? "attending to the *sensus*"?] master of his art, someone says, must apply himself to the body alone and heal pleasantly [*jucunde*]. What can be thought up more pleasant for the cure of the French disease than embracing and enjoying a virgin? But the physician is also, one will have to object, a sensitive master of his art; however, "sensitive" does not mean that he should take into account the body alone and not worry about the soul.[71]

There is no evidence that Sitoni was pointing to Rodrigo a Castro behind his elusive and possibly merely rhetorical *quisquam*, although it is true that in one of his most emphatic definitions of his model physician, Castro had pointed out that the ideal cure should also be pleasant, using the word Sitoni highlights (*jucundus*): "But a prudent, learned, and serious physician always strives for this: that with greatest modesty he cure quickly and pleasantly, and above all safely."[72] It would be absurd to argue that Sitoni is charging Rodrigo a Castro with advocating the presumed remedy for syphilis. In this passage

Sitoni is interested in a larger and more theoretical point, so theoretical in fact that he has to assume for a moment even the hypothetical curing powers of a virgin, an assumption he knows to be false. "Theoretical," of course, does not mean ethereal, nebulous, or removed from praxis. It means that the argument has moved beyond the issue at hand (for the "somebody" certainly is not Sassonia) to an evaluation of important opposing positions that inform a physician's action. With his *cas limite* that balances the worth of man and of woman and takes into consideration both their physical and spiritual health, Sitoni shows convincingly the limitations of such an ethical position as Castro's when it is pushed to its extreme. Against that position, which as he charges takes into account "the body alone," Sitoni holds up a medical practice that is bounded by Roman Catholic ethics as demonstrated by the physician and canonist Zacchia. It would seem that what I provisionally called Sitoni's "feminist" sensibility is a vehicle for this larger argument, although we may have reached the margin of what is provable. With his argument, opposing the secular medicine that seemed dominant at least for some time at Padua and at Hamburg (where Castro wrote all his books), Sitoni fits perfectly into the emerging line of Catholic medical ethicists (close to the Counter-Reformation) from Codronchi through Zacchia to the physician-priest Girolamo Bardi (1600–1667), who had wanted to be a Jesuit.[73] In any case, the opposition between a "secular" medical ethics and a medical practice bounded by traditional religious ethics adumbrates the ideological fault lines that have appeared again in modern discussions of syphilis and AIDS.[74] In the first sections of this chapter we saw that, despite the demise of the particular prescriptions for the care and prevention of syphilis (such as mercury, guaiacum wood, Falloppio's *linteolum*), Renaissance discussions of the prevention of this disease relate to pressing issues of our day. However, the material adduced in the final section may put us on guard against facile homologies, for it now appears that the "secular" and "progressive" medical ethics of Sassonia and Castro could more readily accommodate sexist views of disease and therapy than could the religiously defined ethics (of physicians like Sitoni and Bardi), while today the opposite may be true.

I have to leave to the student of mythology the exploration of how to derive the notion that intercourse with a virgin should have a curative effect. Perhaps in this notion her role is analogous to what in early Greek literature is called the *therápon*, some alter ego onto whom one's impurities may be transferred. (Thus, as Gregory Nagy and others have pointed out, Patroklos functions as *therápon* of Achilles.)[75] More specifically, other ideas about the powers of virginity and even about the powers of the Virgin might be relevant, for at work might be a form of thinking theologians call *recirculatio*, quite common in medieval theology (as, to give one instance, "lost by the tree—saved by the tree," i.e. the tree of paradise versus the tree of the Cross): lost by a woman—saved by a woman.

It may be objected that the two kinds of gender imbalance in relation to syphilis pointed up in this essay, i.e. imputation of blame for venereal infection to women and the notion of male cleansing through intercourse with a virgin, are arcane and recondite. However, the former kind of imbalance seems to cut across a good number of both rational (i.e. Galenic) academic physicians and those willing to draw on Paracelsus; such references could easily be multiplied. As to the antithetical notion that the virgin is capable of healing the syphilitic, I may have exhausted learned documentation or elite discourse on that point with the passages quoted from Scaliger, Sassonia, and Zwinger. But paucity of passages in this field of sexuality, for obvious and demonstrated reasons highly tabooed, does not mean lack of importance. For, to use George Boas's words, it characterizes the proper detachment of the historian of ideas "to treat ideas that seem silly or superstitious and are perhaps obsolete with the same care as [one] would give to established truths. For the history of ideas tells us among other things how we got to think the way we do—and if that is not of importance, one wonders what is."[76]

NOTES

1. Paul Diepgen, *Über den Einfluss der autoritativen Theologie auf die Medizin des Mittelalters* (Wiesbaden: Steiner, 1958 (Akademie der Wissenschaften und der Literatur: Abhandlungen der geistes- und sozialwissenschaftlichen Klasse, 1958; No. 1), p. 8 and *passim*; Owsei Temkin, *The Double Face of Janus and Other Essays in the History of Medicine* (Baltimore and London: Johns Hopkins University Press, 1977), particularly the essays, "Medicine and the Problem of Moral Responsibility," and, "On the History of 'Morality and Syphilis.'" On Francisco Delgardo, see Richmond Cranston Holcomb, *Who Gave the World Syphilis? The Haitian Myth* (New York: Froben, 1937), p. 146. Anthony Grafton with April Shelford and Nancy Siraisi, *New Worlds, Ancient Texts: The Power of Tradition and the Shock of Discovery* (Cambridge, Mass.: Harvard University Press, 1992), p. 193.

2. In his indispensable *Bibliotheca realis medica* (Frankfurt, 1679), pp. 189–93.

3. Ulrich von Hutten, *De guaici medicina et morbo gallico* (Mainz, 1524), c. 2 (sig. b2). For an early trans. see *De morbo Gallico*, trans. Thomas Paynel (London, 1533; STC 14024), fol. 1. For a scholarly translation with valuable footnotes, see Ulrich von Hutten, *Le livre de la maladie française*, ed. F. F. A. Potton (Lyon: Perrin, 1865), p. 17. A facsimile reprint of Leoniceno, *Libellus de epedemia, quam vulgo morbum Gallicum vocant* (Venice, 1497), is included in *The Earliest Printed Literature on Syphilis*, ed. Karl Sudhoff and Charles Singer (Florence: Lier, 1925). The best recent general study addressing the problem of the origin of syphilis and many other matters relating to the disease, which would serve as an ideal background reading for my more narrow study, is Claude Quétel, *History of Syphilis*, trans. Judith Braddock and Brian Pike (London: Polity Press, 1990).

4. Barrough, "The Sixth Booke Containing the Cure of the Disease Called Morbus Gallicus," in *The Methode of Phisicke* (3d. ed., London, 1596), p. 361.

5. Blankaart, *Abhandlung der sogenannten Frantzoss oder Spanischen Pocken-Krankheit*, in his *Die belägert- und entsetzte Venus* (Leipzig, 1689), p. 2.

6. Ibid, pp. 4 and 487, respectively.

7. *De guaiaci medicina*, c.1 (1524 ed., fol. a4^v). *De morbo Gallico*, trans. Paynel fol. 1^v, and Hutten, *livre de la maladie française*, ed. Potton, p. 4. Hutten says that the word derives from a saint whose name he does not know. According to the editor (Potton), this would be Mevius or Menius, invoked against skin diseases. Potton also notes that the physician Laurent Joubert (1529–1583) derives *mevium* from *minnen*, an "obscene word" for the genitals. *Minne* of course means "love." I suggest that there may be a confusion with L. *menium*, usually glossed by L. *vestibulum*, "front room" or "gallery," possibly used for genitals by euphemistic transference.

8. Bullein, "The Booke of Compoundes," fols. 42^v-43, in his *Bulwarke of Defence Against All Sicknesse* (London, 1579); first ed., 1562.

9. Clowes, *A Briefe and Necessarie Treatise Touching the Cure of the Disease Called Morbus Gallicus* (London, 1585), c. 2, fol. 2^v. Johannes Fabricius calls Clowes "the first English venereologist." See Fabricius, *Syphilis in Shakespeare's England* (London and Bristol, Pennsylvania: Jessica Kingsley, 1994), p. 106.

10. See the section "Sin as Sickness" in chap. 3 of my *Imagery of John Donne's Sermons* (Providence, R. I.: Brown University Press, 1970), pp. 68–85.

11. Wither, *Britain's Remembrancer* (London, 1628), fol. 45v.

12. Clowes, *A Prooved Practice, for All Young Chirurgians, Concerning Burnings with Gunpowder. Hereto is adjoyned a Treatise of the French and Spanish Pockes . . . by J. Almenar* (n.p., 1588), p. 111. Almenar's work is of 1502.

13. Rosebury, *Microbes and Morals: The Strange Story of Venereal Disease* (New York: Viking, 1971), p. 122.

14. Von Hutten, (1524 ed.), c.1 fol. a4^v: "Ibi tum Dei iram interpretati sunt Theologi, quem hanc malorum a nobis morum poenam exigere, hoc supplicium sumere, ac si in supernum illud consilium admissi aliquando didicis-

sent, publice docuerunt, quasi nunquam peius vixerint homines. . . ." Ed. Potton, p. 6. In his English translation of 1533 [fol. 1ᵛ-fol. 2], Paynel tones down the ridicule.

15. For a broader treatment of the subject, see Claude Quétel, *History of Syphilis*, particularly the section, "Remedies," pp. 58–63.

16. *The Earliest Printed Literature on Syphilis*, ed. Sudhoff and Singer, Introduction, p. xxxii.

17. *Tractatus, cum consiliis contra pudendagram sive morbum Gallicum*, in *Earliest Printed Literature on Syphilis*, p. 190: "Dicunt Astrologi hunc morbum evenire a constellatione corporum superiorum. Nam dicunt quod effectus universalis in causas universales resolvi debet. Alii dicunt quod est flagellum dei."

18. Ibid., p. 113.

19. Massa, *Il libro del mal francese* (Venice, 1566), p. 279; cf. Quétel, *History of Syphilis*, p. 58.

20. Massa, *Il libro del mal francese*, p. 282: ". . . con il presidio divino (donde derivano tutti i beni)."

21. Estienne, *L'introduction au traitté de la conformité des merveilles anciennes avec les modernes* (Lyon, 1592), bk. 1, chap. 13, p. 86.

22. Gabriele Falloppio, *De morbo Gallico*, in *Opera omnia* (Frankfurt, 1600), vol. 1, 737: "Ego nihil fecisse videor, nisi doceam vos, quomodo quis videns pulcherrimam sirenam, et coiens cum ea, etiam infecta, a carie et lue Gallica praeservetur. Ego semper fui huius sententiae, quod adsitratio praecavendi, ne per contagium huiusmodi ulcera oriantur. Sed quae est ista ratio?" In the Paduan edition of 1564, the passages to which I am referring are pp. 52–53ᵛ.

23. Ibid., vol. 1, p. 737: "Ideo investigavi hoc medicamentum. Sed quia oportet etiam meretricum animos disponere, non licet nobiscum unguenta domo afferrre. Propterea ego inveni linteolum imbutum medicamento, quod potest commode asportari, cum femoralia iam vasta feratis, ut totam apothecam vobiscum habere possitis."

24. Quétel, *History of Syphilis*, p. 59.

25. Falloppio, *De morbo Gallico*, in *Opera omnia*, vol. 1, p. 682: "Hoc est perpetuum et aeternum dogma: quod propter peccatum advenit mors, et propter errorem poena. Hinc factum est, quod Deus saepe morbis castigavit peccata nostra."

26. Ibid., 683: "Causam huius explicandam relinquo Theologis." On the use of the rhetorical figure *praeteritio* in sensitive contexts, see my essay, "Burton's Use of *praeteritio* in Discussing Same-Sex Relationships," in *Renaissance Discourses of Desire*, ed. Claude J. Summers and Ted-Larry Pepworth (Columbia, Mo., and London: University of Missouri Press, 1993), pp. 159–78.

27. Falloppio, *Opera omnia*, vol. 1, 683: "Novissimum est, quod prae manibus habemus, et morbum Gallicum seu Gallicam scabiem appellamus, missum a Deo, ut timidiores facti Veneris luxuriam relinquamus, et studiis non solum literarum, sed etiam bonarum omnium artium incubamus."

28. Ercole Sassonia, *Luis venereae perfectissimus tractatus* (Patavii, 1597): "Remedia iis, qui scortantur ne tam facile lue corripiantur."

29. Rudio, *De morbis occultis et venenatis* (Venice 1610; first ed., 1604), lib. 5, c. 13: "Remedia valida pro praeservatione a Gallica lue."

30. Ibid., p. 168: "Sed tanti sceleris, atque flagitii Deum ultorem habebit."

31. Ibid., p. 192: "In mulieribus vero meritoriis, quas non propter ipsarum sanitatem, sed propter mares operaepretium est praeservare. . . ."

32. Ibid., p. 168: "Hoc pro salute Medicorum praesertim monuisse volui. Nam si turpe est alios decipi, turpissimum erit, si artem Medicam profitentes in salebras inciderint."

33. Daniel Sennert, "Of the French Pox," in Daniel Sennert, Nicholas Culpeper, Abdiah Cole, *Two Treatises. The First of the Venereal Pocks, The Second Treatise of the Gout* (London 1660), p. 27. The Latin version is in *De lue venerea*, c. 1, in Sennert, *Opera omnia* (Lyon, 1666), vol. 4–5, p. 1014.

34. Sennert, "Of the French Pox," in *Two Treatises*, p. 27.

35. Aurelio Minadoi, *Tractatus de virulentia venerea* (Venice, 1596).

36. Ibid., chap. 31, pp. 164–65.

37. Julien Le Paumier, *De morbis contagiosis* (Paris, 1578), lib. 1, c. 9, p. 37: "Quae cum ita se habeant, si cui luem veneream declinare est animus, eum vel in totum ab impuro concubitu, alioque venereo attactu abstinere, quod Christianos omno decet, vel ita corpus praeparare ac praemunire opportet ut eam minime admittat."

38. August Hirsch's standard biographical dictionary of important physicians in history has no vital dates for Minadoi. (*Biographisches Lexikon der hervorragenden Ärzte aller Zeiten*, 2d ed. [Berlin: Urban und Schwarzenberg, 1929–34]).

39. Allan M. Brandt has described in detail the similarity between attitudes toward syphilis and toward AIDS, and an editorial in the same issue of *Science* speaks of conflicts arising from "the clash of pragmatism and morality." Brandt, "The Syphilis Epidemic and Its Relationship to AIDS," *Science* 239 (1988): 375–80; for the editorial, p. 539. As to attitudes toward AIDS, Harvey V. Fineberg calls the opposing sides somewhat debatably "moralist" and "rationalist": "There is a fundamental disagreement about the propriety of educational messages to prevent AIDS. . . . For some the only socially acceptable change is to have people altogether abandon certain behaviors. In this moralist view, it is wrong to have sexual relations outside marriage and it is wrong to use drugs, hence it is wrong to advocate or even discuss anything (such as the use of condoms or sterile needles) that would appear to condone these activities. Others take what might be called a rationalist view: behaviors that will occur and are dangerous should be modified so as to make them safer. Such philosophical differences underlie the reticence of many national leaders about AIDS education, controversies about the propriety of specific educational materials. . . ." Fineberg, "Education to Prevent AIDS: Prospects and Obstacles," *Science* 239 (1988): 592–96, particularly p. 593.

40. See my essay, "Renaissance Moralizing of Syphilis and Moral Issues about Prevention," *Bulletin of the History of Medicine* 68 (1994): 389–410.

41. Anna Foa, "The New and the Old: The Spread of Syphilis (1494–1530)," in *Sex and Gender in Historical Perspective: Selections from Quaderni*

Storici, ed. Edward Muir and Guido Ruggiero (Baltimore and London: Johns Hopkins University Press, 1990), pp. 26–45.

42. See Karl Figlio, "Chlorosis and Chronic Disease in 19th-Century Britain: The Social Construction of Somatic Illness in a Capitalist Society," in *Women and Health: The Politics of Sex in Medicine,* ed. Elizabeth Fee (Farmingdale, N.Y.: Baywood, 1983), pp. 231–41; and Gerald M. Oppenheimer, "In the Eye of the Storm: The Epidemiological Construction of AIDS," in *AIDS: The Burdens of History,* ed. Elizabeth Fee and Daniel M. Fox (Berkeley: University of California Press, 1988), pp. 267–300. On the construction of human sexology through the ages, see Thomas W. Laqueur, *Making Sex: Body and Gender from the Greeks to Freud* (Cambridge, Mass.: Harvard University Press, 1990). Anthony Grafton and others, *New Worlds, Ancient Texts,* p. 188. My discussion follows closely my essay, "Infection and Cure through Women: Renaissance Constructions of Syphilis," *Journal of Medieval and Renaissance Studies,* 24 (1994): 501–17.

43. *Method of Physicke,* 3d ed., p. 373.

44. *Luis venereae perfectissimus tractatus,* fol. 5v: ". . . ex nimia vulvae caliditate."

45. "Some Curious Problems . . . Concerning the Venereal Distemper," in *A New Method of Curing the French-Pox* (London, 1690), p. 121 (Wing N672).

46. On the history of female sexuality, see Danielle Jacquart and Claude Thomasset, *Sexuality and Medicine in the Middle Ages,* trans. M. Adamson (Princeton, N.J.: Princeton University Press, 1985); Ian Maclean, *The Renaissance Notion of Woman: A Study in the Fortunes of Scholasticism and Medieval Science in European Intellectual Life* (Cambridge: Cambridge University Press, 1985). Specifically, on England, see Audrey Eccles, *Obstetrics and Gynaecology in Tudor and Stuart England* (Kent, Ohio: Kent State University Press, 1982); and Patricia Crawford, "Attitudes to Menstruation in Seventeenth-Century England," *Past and Present* 91 (1981): 47–73. On a related subject, Ottavia Niccoli, "'Mentruum Quasi Monstrum': Monstrous Births and Menstrual Taboo in the Sixteenth Century," in *Sex and Gender in Historical Perspective,* pp. 1–25.

47. Rostino, *Trattato di mal francese* (Venice, 1556), pp. 28–36; Torrella, *Tractatus cum consiliis contra pudendagram seu morbum Gallicum* (1497), in *The Earliest Printed Literature on Syphilis.*

48. Héry, *La méthode curatoire de la maladie vénérienne* (Paris, 1660), p. 2. On Héry, see Quétel, *History of Syphilis,* p. 62.

49. Parcelsus, *Chirurgia magna* (Strasbourg, 1573; first ed., 1536), p. 97, reported by Anna Foa, "The New and the Old," in *Sex and Gender in Historical Perspective,* p. 39.

50. Blankaart (1650–1702), *Abhandlung der sogenannten Franzoss oder Spanischen Pocken-Krankheit,* in his *Die belägert und entsetzte Venus,* p. 4.

51. Paracelsus, *Sämtliche Werke,* ed. Karl Sudhoff, vol. 7 (München: Barth, 1923), p. 189, and *Opera omnia* (Geneva, 1658), vol. 2, p. 174.

52. Mattioli, in *Morbi Gallici curandi ratio equisitissima a variis . . . medicis conscripta,* ed. Joseph Tectander (Basel, 1536), p. 8: "Nonnulli morbum Gallos, cum per montem Salvium iter facerent, a foeminis leprosis per coitum primitus contraxisse, eorum postea intemperantia atram bilem pituitamque procurante, memoriae prodiderunt."

53. See my essay, "Le feu caché: Homosocial Bonds Between Women in a Renaissance Romance," *Renaissance Quarterly* 45 (1992): 293–311.

54. Vives, *The Instruction of a Christian Woman* (n.p., 1541), fol. 74–77 (STC 24858), and "De institutione foeminae christianae," lib. 2, c. 4, in Vives, *Opera* (Basel, 1555), vol. 2, pp. 707–08.

55. Theodor Zwinger, *Theatrum vitae humanae* (Basel [1604]), 374a. As to the stage of Bernard's syphilis when he married, he was most likely not infectious. Therefore it is consistent with the usual course of the disease that Clara remained uninfected for twenty years and had nonluetic children.

56. Carlos G. Noreña, *Juan Luis Vives* (The Hague: Nijhoff, 1970; International Archives of the History of Ideas, no. 34), p. 51.

57. In the context of writing on women as innocent victims, Anthony Grafton mentions Erasmus and Alciati: See Grafton and others, *New Worlds, Ancient Texts*, p. 188. Geoffrey Whitney, *A Choice of Emblemes* (Leiden, 1586), p. 99, takes over the emblem with the Erasmian lemma: *Impar coniugium.*

58. Sassonia, *Luis venereae tractatus*, c. 37, fol. 40: "Sciendum autem est, quod habui a quibusdam expertis Venetis; Dicunt se a Gonorrhaea statim curatos usu Veneris cum mulier Aethiope. Experimentum est verum, et videtur posse confirmari ex Scaligero exercitatione 180. cap. 18. qui scribit Affros a Lue Venerea curari, dum in Numidam, et Aethiopam sucedunt. Haec quoque scio, si tamen literis consignam licet antiqua gonorrhaea plures fuisse liberatos, qui cum uxore Virgine rem habuerunt, sed tunc mulier inficitur."

59. Scaliger, *Exotericarum Exercitationum liber XV de subtilitate*, exercitatio 181, c. 19 (Hannover, 1620), p. 563: "Qui eo laborant, si in Numidiam aut in Nigricam sese conferant Aethiopiam, solius Caeli beneficio, sine ullis medicamentis convalescere." On attributing syphilis to the Jew as the "other," see Anna Foa, "The New and The Old," in *Sex and Gender in Historical Perspective.*

60. Sitoni, *Miscellanea medico-curiosa* (2d ed., Cologne, 1677), tractatus 45.

61. Ibid., p. 288: "Sed non a foeminis solum in masculos pertransit, cum reciprocus sit et a masculis in foeminas etiam transferatur."

62. Ibid.: "Nihilominus remedium quoddam huius labis celebratur ab aliquibus tanquam ad infectorum virorum curationem certissimum."

63. Ibid., p. 293: "Haec quoque scio, si tamen litteris consignem: scilicet ab antiqua gonorrhaea plures fuisse liberatos, qui cum uxore virgine rem habuerunt, sed tunc mulier inficitur."

64. Ibid., p. 294: ". . . concludunt non solum Canonistae omnes, sed et Medici catholice sentientes."

65. Zacchia, *Questiones medico-legales* (3d ed., Amsterdam, 1651), lib. 6, tit. 1, q. 5, p. 380.

66. Ibid.: "Ego quidem non modo existemaverim peccare Medicum conditionaliter loquentem, ut Navarra dicit, Ego tibi non consulo, sed si tale quid faceres, sanareris, sed etiamsi cum haec exceptione loqueretur, Nisi peccatum obstaret, coitus usus tibi sanitatem restitueret."

67. Sitoni, *Miscellanea*, p. 296: "Suadet temporis opportunitas, quae bacchanalia concedit iis, quos praesentis belli calamitas lugere non facit."

68. Sassonia, *Luis venerae tractatus* fol. 4: "Altera vero fuit Nicoleta meretrix Venetiis notissima, quae cum iam annos quatuor continuos Hectica Venerea laborasset, ac per id tempus semper decubuisset, ligni Indici decocto sanitati est restituta, ita ut hoc etiam tempore iterum artem mereticam profiteatur."

69. Castro, *Medicus-Politicus* (Hamburg, 1614), p. 138. The chapter (lib. 3, c. 8) is entitled, "How far should the patient's wishes be gratified?"

70. "Philaletes Lusitanus," otherwise unknown, in a prefatory letter to Benedict a Castro, *Flagellum calumniantium* (Amsterdam, 1631). Benedict (or Baruch) is Rodrigo a Castro's son, also a successful physician. On Rodrigo a Castro, see Harry Friedenwald, *Jews in Medicine: Essays*, 2 vols. (Baltimore: Johns Hopkins University Press, 1944), vol. 2, pp. 448–49: "The Doctors de Castro." On the embattled status of expatriate Portuguese Jews in Renaissance Central Europe, see R. Bandeira, "La Renaissance et l'Ecole Iatroéthique Portugaise du XVIᵉ siècle," in *Atti, XXI Congresso internationale di Storia della Medicina* (*1988*), ed. Raffaele A. Bernabeo (Bologna: Monduzzi, 1988), pp. 675–81, and my essay, "Renaissance Medical Ethics: The Contribution of Exiled Portuguese Jews," in *Expulsion of the Jews:* (*1492*), ed. R. B. Waddington and A. H. Williamson (New York and London: Garland, 1994), pp. 147–59.

71. Sitoni, *Miscellanea*, p. 294: "Oportet, quod Medicus, qui est artifex sensitivus (dicit quisquam) soli corpori incumbat, et iucunde medeatur. Ad quid jucundus ad morbi Gallici curationem excogitari potest, quam virginis amplexus, concubitus. Est equidem (respondebitur) Medicus artifex sensitivus; sed non ita sensitivus, ut solius corporis rationem habere debeat, ac de anima solicitus non sit."

72. Castro, *Medicus-Politicus*, lib. 3, c. 24 (p. 205): "Cordatus vero, eruditus, et gravis medicus id semper ante oculos habet, ut summa modestia cito et iucunde, presertim vero tuto, curet."

73. Battista Codronchi, *De Christiana et tuta medendi ratione* (Ferrara 1591) and Bardi, *Medicus politico Catholicus* (Genua, 1644). Bardi left the Society for health reasons.

74. See n. 39. See also Elizabeth Fee, "Sin versus Science: Venereal Disease in 20th-Century Baltimore," in *AIDS: The Burden of History*, ed. Elizabeth Fee and Daniel M. Fox (Berkeley: University of California Press, 1988), pp. 121–46.

75. Nagy, *The Best of the Achaeans: Concepts of the Hero in Archaic Greek Poetry* (Baltimore and London: Johns Hopkins University Press, 1979), p. 292.

76. Boas, *The History of Ideas* (New York: Scribner's, 1969), p. viii.

Conclusion

The works considered in this study are by medical authors writing roughly between the 1550s and 1650s and include books on the duties of physicians, collections of cases and similar medical genres, and books on medical practice. I screened the last group particularly with respect to women's diseases and the treatment of syphilis. Then, as now, medical ethics was a terrain of ideological minefields. Today we wonder what is the relationship of bioethics to moral theology, to "natural law," or to the majority vote of the electorate. Or what should be the credentials of persons professing medical ethics? Likewise, in the century studied, when something like an incipient field of medical ethics was constituting itself, there were also dangerous ideological quicksands. Sometimes the fault lines, to vary the metaphor, are gaping, sometimes they are concealed or tenuously bridged. The impression one gets is not that ethical questions were considered a frill, hobby, or occasional subject for Sunday meditation, but that they deeply involved the entire being and practice of the physicians: not only their relationship to patients and *adstantes* but also to their colleagues and to powerful institutions of church and state. For Rodrigo a Castro to clarify his moral duties in these various respects was, from one perspective, merely a *lusus senectutis*, a game of old age, as he once put it somewhat aristocratically, but from another it was a deeply probing investigation and an undertaking hardly ever attempted before. If some of my analysis is correct, such clarification was essential for his professional survival: it was not only a validation of his profession but a public defense of his personal commitment to medicine.

In the second chapter we saw that in the Renaissance, medical ruse or deception becomes for some physicians, most notably Alessandrini and Castro, a topic discussed in its own right—ancient medicine had supplied only a few bare hints. The problem of how to decide when one is morally justified in withholding information from the patient, a problem on which the Renaissance had more elaborate and firm opinions than the ancients, is one of the issues that modern medical ethicists still think should be in the curriculum of each medical school.[1] In the Renaissance, this prehistory of the effects of autosuggestion (including placebo effects) ranged from withholding information ("dissimulation" in the old and precise sense) to active deception ("simulation").

The most ingenious stratagems for curing by ruse as well as the most probing ethical discussions of medical deception appear to originate from the Iberian peninsula. While a clear fault line between Catholic and Protestant positions on this issue cannot be demonstrated, there are other demarcations: the difference between, on the one hand, an Iberian physician solving a moral dilemma (the question whether to cooperate with a patient in a certain kind of deception) by seeking advice from the moral-theological expert and, on the other, the French professor of medicine claiming in a similar case that his decision whether to cooperate or not falls within the purview of the medical doctor and not the priest; and the difference between accounts of deception in equivalent books on medical duties by someone publicly committed to Catholicism (possibly a New Christian) and by someone who at one time or another would have been considered a Marrano and "Judaizer." (Reshaping a biblical story, Henriques, on the way to professorships in philosophy and medicine in the most prestigious universities of Spain and Portugal, writes a disquisition against any form of deceit, while Castro, with the help of classical learning, sides with the practice of classical and recent medicine in justifying ruses in the interest of cure.)

In the fourth chapter, we contrasted the secular position that Castro had developed in defending himself against Christian detractors with important Roman Catholic writers on medical ethics. Most of the differences (but not all) go back to fundamentally different views about the physician's work in relation to body and soul. In the "Public Letter" (*Epistola nuncupatoria*) that opened his often-quoted book on Christian medical ethics, *De Christiana ac tuta medendi ratione*, the Roman Catholic physician Codronchi had programmatically outlined the nexus (*coniunctio*) between mind and body and their reciprocal influence, a topic eminently important to physicians on all parts of the Catholic spectrum, from the more moderate Codronchi to the physician-priest Bardi. Since, as he put it, the "sympathy" between body and soul was so close that the vices of the mind (*animi vitia*) influenced the body and, in turn, bodily diseases weakened the mind, Codronchi "was forced to affirm that physicians undertake not only the cure of the body, which is the coarser part of man, but also that of the mind."[2] Codronchi sees theologians and physicians working for the same aim: physical and mental health. In this context, Codronchi adds a strikingly simple and memorable distinction, apparently passing it off as his own, although it is not: "The theologians take the soul as a starting point, while the physicians begin with the body."[3]

In fact, this had been a key phrase in Erasmus's "Praise of Medicine," a praise possibly overblown, as is indicated by the generic term Erasmus used for the piece, *declamatio*, i.e. an exercise in epideixis. The famous humanist's praise included the argument that physicians by their therapy not only effectively determined whether a patient was melancholic or possessed but (considerably more daringly) that physicians, by reestablishing the balance of the humors, made diabolic possession unlikely or even impossible; this point had in some sense become part of medical literature—Jérôme Monteux, for instance, includes Erasmus's entire piece in his books on medicine.[4] This was probably as far as one could extend the physician's territory within the traditional dualistic pneumatology of the Roman Catholic church. (John Henry points out that the dualism is essentially the same in the major Reformed churches).[5] Beyond that position, from the traditional viewpoint, was the abyss of monistic philosophy, seen as subversive and irreligious.

Would Rodrigo a Castro have agreed with Codronchi's view (derived from Erasmus)? As we saw, Castro does not mention Codronchi's important work on medical ethics, although he cites another work by the same author. Taken literally, Codronchi's entire collection of ethical principles would have made the medical profession impossible for Castro, and Castro's *Medicus-Politicus* is expressedly conceived as an alternative or fresh start on thinking through the duties of the physician. The Christian churches' well-known dogmatic positions about body and soul may not have made it seem inviting for Castro to redefine his stand, although he demonstrates at every juncture that his emphasis is on curing the body rather than the soul. While, compared with Codronchi, he stresses naturalistic ways of treating illness, it was up to his Lusitani (i.e. Portuguese-Jewish) defenders to harden this position to a cure of *only* the body while denying any impact of the physician on the soul. In general Castro anticipates the position that John Henry, in his important essay on the cultural landscape in England, sees as characteristic of the second half of the seventeenth century: "Thus, at a time when many believed that sickness was visited upon mankind by God, the physician was seen everywhere as ignoring such religious considerations and treating sickness in an entirely naturalistic way" (p. 89).

As we saw, Castro is silent on *De Christiana ac tuta medendi ratione*. When he speaks out against a near-contemporary writer on medical ethics, it is on an issue without clear dogmatic signposts: the medical treatment of enemies. Castro's sharp disagreement is motivated by the strong humanistic sense that animates all his work as a physician. I have argued that this sense may have been generated both by his experience of partially overcoming his difficulties of "otherness" in his elective city and by the voices of detractors fomenting antipathy against Jewish physicians. As he put it in the preface to his *Medicus-Politicus*, "even if the physician is troubled by a person raving, he should not for that matter deny the patient medication."[6] His disagreement with Alessandrini, a Christian physician, on the issue of the medical treatment of enemies may be so unusually sharp because Christians tended to speak as if they owned the virtue of charity. (Castro's son Benedict [or Baruch] was to poke fun at the narrowness of the Christian doctors' self-perception in this respect.) In the matter of charity and in the name of the principle of *humanitas*, Castro was here passing the Christian physician as it were on the inside track. Based on a clever re-reading of (pseudo-)Hippocrates, on the medical example of his Portuguese (and Jewish) uncle, and on his own experience, his plea for physicians to stretch out a hand to the enemy becomes a ringing plea for that secularized virtue of *humanitas*.

Important as is Castro's disagreement with Alessandrini and others on the issue of the medical treatment of enemies, attitudes about the duality of body and soul are of a more fundamental order. Although it might appear that a Salamanca-trained physician like Castro would have no objection in principle to the Erasmian dictum (co-opted by Codronchi) that the physician starts from the body while the theologian starts from the soul, based as that view is on traditional dualistic pneumatology, I am inclined to think that ultimately Castro and Codronchi represent *in statu nascendi* fundamentally different positions in medical ethics. Castro adumbrates the position, so strong in the later centuries, that rests cultural authority and jurisdiction with physicians (and ultimately clinicians), while Codronchi sees medical ethics as cohering with the larger cultural and religious belief systems, a position powerfully represented today by the books of such thinkers as John M. Frame, Bernhard Häring, and John T. Noonan.

But such classification, which tends to shed all the specificity of the previous centuries, is of only limited help. If pressed too hard, it becomes anachronistic and an example of the worst kind of medical history, namely the one interested merely in identifying forerunners of presumed present achievements and positions. Aware of such fallacies, I therefore (in the fifth chapter) deliberately tried to listen to what physicians in the early seventeenth century singled out as important in medical ethics in their time. The result may strike some readers as strange indeed. When I read a section of chapter 5 at a major medical research institution, a scholar working in modern bioethics could not recognize the overlap of subject between my theme and his. The subtext of his remark seemed to be that the moral dilemma about treating a particular version of what was called "hysteria," because it was based on outdated reproductive physiology, is too arcane to be instructive today. My answer was that when a physician writes in 1612 that a certain dilemma is the most difficult problem in the medicine of his day, historians, bioethicists, and even physicians need to listen.

The problem of removing female and male seed led us to notions about gender in areas where Renaissance physicians labored with restrictions and taboos different from those of the ancients. In gynecology, all the Roman Catholic thinkers of the later Renaissance that I surveyed except one, while carefully weighing both sides of the issue, finally oppose a procedure recommended by Galen. (In the remaining author, a moral casuist, not a physician, the relevant passages are removed in later editions, possibly after his death.) Since I find no opposition to the therapy before the late sixteenth century, this is one area where a greater sensitivity to ethical matters in the wake of the Reformation and Counter-Reformation can be shown. In another phase of the controversy, Cortesi, risen from barber to surgeon to physician and professor of medicine, and drawing on his expertise in anatomizing, takes to task both parties of the disputants and, finding both wrong, assigns even greater culpability to the physicians, since they ought to know better. What we see played out in miniature is a version of the modern stance in medical ethics according to which superior science would distinguish the more creditable practitioner: belief in the elitism of expertise as cultural authority.

On any scale, the issue raised about putative ways of strengthening the male organs of children will be just as arcane as the gynecological problem mentioned—it belongs to the same field of matters unmentionable in the vernacular: Latin prose, in this instance fraught with stylistic signals like *praeteritio* and denials of immoral intentions, still supplies the appropriate intermediate region in which the otherwise inexpressible is sayable. Careful reading of relevant medical texts of the period, including texts by Falloppius, suggests that they have been misinterpreted by modern historians: I find no evidence that juvenile masturbation was recommended or tolerated. As for adult masturbation, whoever in the Renaissance comments on the relevant passages in Galen—and this includes staunch defenders of the ancient doctor in other matters—does so with disapproval. The Renaissance sensitivity to the issue of masturbation in general and masturbation of children in particular may be in part a reaction to perceived links with homosexuality—and so astute a medical ethicist on many topics as Johann Heinrich Meibom is also evidence that (for a number of reasons)[7] homophobia was especially pronounced in Protestant regions. Thus even this seemingly arcane medical issue is linked to some topics receiving special attention from historians and cultural anthropologists today. At the same time Meibom, city physician of Lübeck, demonstrates that with regard to sexuality, Protestantism does not mean all-pervasive prudery: for at the margin of accepted sexual practices, the Lutheran doctor justifies even flogging as sexual stimulus if it leads to marital intercourse.

My final chapter, with its account of moral issues relating to syphilis in the period, needs no apology for arcaneness, since the modern reader will be thoroughly familiar with the kind of problems discussed. Whether I refer to AIDS or not, the reader will at each juncture of the account, particularly with respect to prevention, have made the connection. I would argue that this is so primarily because a parallel exists through a similarity of the cultural forces at work, and not because modern concerns have determined my treatment. Here, as in several other areas of medical ethics that I mention, the period under discussion appears decidedly "early modern" rather than Renaissance in the important way in which that nomenclature has recently been used by theorists interested in redrawing literary and historical boundaries.[8] But it is true here too that elements that are arcane now and (from the point of view of modern science) mistaken, like the specially prepared post-phylactic *linteolum* advocated by Falloppius, stimulated the most far-reaching ethical discussion then.

This holds true also for an element of therapy already at that time identified as medical mythology: the alleged cure of syphilis by sleeping with a virgin. While some of Sitoni's motives for writing his vigorous critique of that claim remain obscure, his ostensible purpose is to strike a blow at the notion that the physician can cure happily, quickly, and safely without being deeply concerned with his patient's health of mind or the state of his soul. He wants to justify the role of ethics in medicine, an endeavor we recognize in this case as an apology for a specific kind of medical ethics. This is a Roman Catholic ethics, and the argument draws its power from confronting views and practices that are not only gendered but misogynist.

NOTES

1. See C. M. Culver, K. D. Clouser, B. Gert, et al, "Basic Curricular Goals in Medical Ethics," *New England Journal of Medicine,* 312 (1985): 253–56.

2. Codronchi, "Epistola nuncupatoria": "Affirmare debemus, medicos non tantum corporis, quae vilior est hominis pars, verum etiam animi curam suscipere. . . ."

3. Ibid., "Theologi ab animo, Medici vero a corpore sumant initium."

4. Monteux [or Montuus], *Selecta aliquot in aphorismos redacta,* in *Opuscula iuvenilia* (Lyon, 1556), p. 36: "Neque vero corporis tantum, quae vilior hominis pars est, curam gerit, imo totius hominis curam agit, etiamsi Theologus ab animo, medicus a copore sumet initium." Cf. Brian McGregor's translation in Erasmus, *Collected Works,* vol. 29, ed. E. Fantham and E. Rummel (Toronto: University of Toronto Press, 1989), p. 39: "Now the physician is concerned not only with the care of the body, the lower element in man, but with the treatment of the entire man, and just as the theologian takes the soul as a starting-point, the physician begins with the body."

5. John Henry, "The Matter of Souls: Medical Theory and Theology in Seventeenth-Century England," in *The Medical Revolution of the Seventeenth Century,* ed. Roger French and Andrew Wear (Cambridge: Cambridge University Press, 1989), pp. 87–113; particularly p. 88.

6. *Medicus-Politius,* Sig. A2v: "Molestus est medicus furenti: non tamen propterea neganda est infirmo medicina."

7. See my essay, "'That Matter Which Ought Not To Be Heard Of': Homophobic Slurs in Renaissance Cultural Politics," *Journal of Homosexuality* 26 (1994): 41–75.

8. See Leah S. Marcus, "Renaissance/Early Modern Studies," in *Redrawing the Boundaries: The Transformation of English and American Literary Studies,* ed. Stephen Greenblatt and Giles Gunn (New York: The Modern Language Association of America, 1992), pp. 41–63.

Bibliography

Primary Sources

Alexandrinus, Julius. *De medicina et medico*. Zürich, 1557.

Almenar, Juan. *Libellus ad evitandum et expellendum morbum gallicum ut nunquam revertatur noviter inventus ac impressus. . . .* Venice, 1502.

Antoninus, Saint. *Summa theologica*. Lyon, 1542.

Argenterio, Giovanni. *De consultationibus medicis sive (ut vulgus vocat) de collegiandi ratione liber*. Florence, 1551.

Arnald of Villanova. *De cautelis medicorum*. Trans. Henry E. Sigerist. In *A Source Book of Medieval Science*, ed. Edward Grant. Cambridge, Mass.: Harvard University Press, 1974.

Azor, Juan. *Institutiones morales*. 2 vols. Rome, 1600–06.

Bardi, Girolamo. *Medicus politico Catholicus*. Genua, 1644.

Barrough, Philip. *Methode of Phisicke*. 1583 and 1590. 3d ed., 1596.

Blankaart, Stephen. *Abhandlung der sogenannten Frantzoss oder Spanischen Pocken-Krankheit*. In *Die belägert- und entsetzte Venus*. Leipzig, 1689.

Botallo, Leonardo. *Commentarioli duo, alter de medici, alter de aegroti munere*. Lyon, 1565.

Bottoni, Albertino. *De morbis muliebribus*. Libri tres. Venice, 1588.

Boudewyns, Michel. *Ventilabrum medico-theologicum*. Antwerp, 1666.

Bullein, William. *Bulwarke of Defence Against all Sicknesse*. London, 1579.

Carera, Antonio. *Le confusioni de medici. Opera nella quale si scuopono gl'error, e gl'inganni de Medici*. Milano, 1652.

Castelli, Pietro. *Optimus medicus*. Messanae, 1637.

———. *De visitatione aegrotantium. Pro suis auditoribus et discipulis ad praxim instruendis*. Rome, 1630.

Castro, Benedict a. *Flagellum calumniantium*. Amsterdam, 1631.

Castro, Rodrigo a. *Medicus-Politicus*. Hamburg, 1614.

———. *De universa mulierum medicina*. Hamburg, 1603.

Clowes, William. *A Briefe and Necessarie Treatise Touching the Cure of the Disease Called Morbus Gallicus*. London, 1585.

———. *A Prooved Practice, for All Young Chirurgians, Concerning Burnings with Gunpowder. Hereto is adjoyned a Treatise of the French and Spanish Pockes . . . by J. Almenar*. London, 1591. 1st ed., 1588.

Codronchi, Battista. *De Christiana ac tuta medendi ratione*. Ferrara, 1591.

———. *De morbis veneficis, et veneficiis libri IV*. Milan, 1618; 1st ed., 1595.

————. *De rabie, hydrophobia communiter dicta.* Frankfurt, 1610.

————. *De vitiis vocis.* Frankfurt, 1597.

Colle, Giovanni. *Cosmitor medicaeus.* Venice, 1621.

La *Continuation du Mercure françois ou Suitte de l'Histoire de l'Auguste Régence de la Royne Marie de Medicis, sous son fils . . . Louis XIII.* Paris, 1613.

Corbeius, Hermann. *Gynaeceium.* Frankfurt, 1620.

Cornarius, Jeremias. *Fori medici adumbratio.* Coburg, 1607.

Cortesi, Giovanni Battista. *Miscellaneorum medicinalium decades.* Messanae, 1625.

Culpeper, Nicholas, Abdiah Cole, and William Rowland. *The Practice of Physick. Being chiefly a Translation of the Works of Lazarus Reverius.* London, 1672.

Curtius, Joachim. *Exhortatio inclytae rei publicae, cur Judaei a congressu conversatione et praxi Medicorum arcendi sint.* Hamburg, 1632.

Donati, Marcello. *De medica historia mirabili.* 1586.

Dubois, Jacques. *De mensibus mulierum, et hominis generatione.* In *Gynaeciorum sive de mulierum affectibus commentiarii Graecorum, Latinorum, Barbarorum.* Ed. Caspar Wolphius. Basel, 1587.

Duret, Louis. *Commentary in Jacques Houllier, Opera omnia practica L. Dureti annotationibus.* Geneva, 1623.

Erasmus. *Collected Works.* Vol. 29. Ed. E. Fantham and E. Rummel. Trans. Brian McGregor. Toronto: University of Toronto Press, 1989.

Estienne, Henri. *L'introduction au traitté de la conformité des merveilles anciennes avec les modernes.* Lyon, 1592.

Falloppio, Gabriele. *Opera omnia.* Frankfurt, 1600.

Fidele, Fortunato. *De relationibus medicorum.* Palermo, 1602.

Fienus, Thomas. *De viribus imaginationis.* Leyden, 1635 [1st ed., 1608].

Fontecha, Juan-Alonso de los Ruyzes de. *Medicorum incipientium medicina, sive medicinae Christianae speculum.* [Alcalá], 1598.

Foreest, Peter. *Observationum et curationum medicinalium libri.* Lugduni Batavorum, 1599.

Galen. *Omnia quae exstant.* Basel, 1561.

————. *Opera omnia.* 20 vols. Ed. Karl Gottlob Kühn. Leipzig, 1821–33.

————. *On the Affected Parts.* Trans. Rudolph E. Siegel. Basel: Karger, 1976.

Gerhard, Johann. *Centuria quaestionum politicarum.* 2d ed. Jena, 1608.

Golius, Theophilus. *Epitome doctrina moralis, ex decem libris Ethicorum Aristotelis ad Nichomachum collecta.* Cambridge, 1634.

Grado, Giovanni Matteo da. *Praxis in nonum Almansoris.* Lyon, 1527.

Guainerio, Antonio. *Opera omnia.* Pavia, 1481.

Henriques, Henrique Jorge. *Retrato del perfecto médico.* Salamanca, 1595.

Héry, Thierry de. *La méthode curatoire de la maladie vénérienne.* Paris, 1660.

Heywood, Thomas. *Gynaikeion: or, Nine Bookes of Various History. Concerning Women.* London, 1624.

Hippocrates. *Oeuvres complètes.* Ed. Emile Littré. 10 vols. Paris: Baillière, 1839–61.

————. *Opera omnia quae extant in VIII sectiones . . . distributa.* Frankfurt, 1595.

———. *Pseudoepigraphic Writings.* Ed. and trans. Wesley D. Smith. Leiden and New York: Brill, 1990.

Hörnigk, Ludwig von. *Medicaster Apella oder Juden Artzt.* Strassburg, 1631.

———. *Politia medica.* Frankfurt, 1638.

Huarte de San Juan, Juan. *The Examination of Mens Wits.* Trans. R[ichard] C[arew]. London, 1594.

Hutten, Ulrich von. *De guaiaci medicina et morbo gallico.* Mainz, 1524.

———. *De morbo gallico.* Trans. Thomas Paynel. London, 1533.

———. *Le livre de la maladie francaise.* Ed. F. F. A. Potton. Lyon: Perrin, 1865.

Hyginus. *Fabularum liber.* Basel, 1535.

———. *The Myths of Hyginus.* Trans. and ed. Mary Grant. Lawrence, Kans.: University of Kansas Press, 1960.

Ingrassia, Giovanni Filippo. *Iatrapologia.* Venice, ca. 1550.

Jorden, Edward. *Brief Discourse of a Disease Called the Suffocation of the Mother.* London, 1603.

Joubert, Laurent. *Erreurs populaires au fait de la medicine et régime de santé.* Bordeaux, 1578.

The Key to Unknowne Knowledge. London, 1599.

Kornmann, Heinrich. *Sybyla Tryg Andriana, seu De Virginitate, virginum statu et iure tractatus.* Frankfurt, 1610.

Lapide, Cornelius a. *In libros Regum et Paralipomenon commentarius.* Paris, 1642.

Leoniceno, Nicolò. *Libellus de epidemia, quam vulgo morbum Gallicum vocant.* Venice, 1497.

Le Paumier, Julien. *De morbis contagiosis.* Paris, 1578.

Lipen, Martin. *Bibliotheca realis medica.* Frankfurt, 1679.

Luther, Martin. *Colloquia.* In *Werke.* Weimar: Böhlau, 1883—.

———. *On the Jews and Their Lies.* . . . 1543.

Margarita, Antonius. *Der gantz jüdish Glaub.* [Augsburg], 1530.

Martini, Jacob. *Apella medicaster bullatus oder Judenarzt.* Hamburg, 1636.

Marzio, Galeotto. *De doctrina promiscua.* Lyon, 1552.

Massa, Nicolò. *Il libro del mal francese.* Venice, 1566.

Mattioli, Pietro Andrea. *Apologia adversus Amatum Lusitanum cum censura in eiusdem enarratione.* In *Opera omnia.* Frankfurt, 1608.

———. *Morbi Gallici curandi ratio exquisitissima a variis . . . medicis conscripta.* Ed. Joseph Tectander. Basel, 1536.

Meibomius, Johann Heinrich. *De flagrorum usu in re medica et venerea.* Lugduni Batavorum, 1643.

———. *De flagrorum usu in re venerea.* Paris, 1792.

———. *Horkos, sive jusjurandum.* Leyden, 1643.

———. *A Treatise of the Use of Flogging in Venereal Affairs: Also of the Office of the Loins and Reins.* London, 1718.

Melanchthon. *Ethicae doctrinae elementa.* Wittenberg, 1550.

———. *Philosophia moralis epitomes.* Strassburg, 1542.

Mercado, Luis. *De mulierum affectionibus libri quatuor.* Valladolid, 1597.

———. *Opera.* Frankfurt, 1620.

Mercure françois. Quatriesme tôme, ou Les mémoires de la suitte de l'Histoire de notre temps. Paris, 1617.

Mercuriale, Girolamo. *De morbis muliebribus.* Venice, 1587.

———. *Pisanae praelectiones. In Epidemicas Hippocratis historias.* Venice, 1597.

Minadoi, Aurelio. *Tractatus de virulentia venerea.* Venice, 1596.

Molanus, Johannes. *Medicorum ecclesiasticum diarium.* Louvain, 1595.

Monteux, Jérôme. *Selecta aliquot in aphorismos redacta.* In *Opuscula iuvenilia.* Lyon, 1556.

Moxius, Juan Rafael. *De methodo medendi per venae sectionem morbos muliebres acutos.* Geneva, 1612.

A New Method of Curing the French-Pox. London, 1690. (Wing N672).

Obicius, Hippolitus. *De nobilitate medici contra illius obtrectatores. Dialogus tripartitus.* Venice, 1606.

Paracelsus. *Chirurgia magna.* Strasbourg, 1573. 1st ed., 1536.

———. *Opera omnia.* Geneva, 1658.

———. *Sämtliche Werke.* 1. Abteilung. Ed. Karl Sudhoff. München: Barth, 1923.

Paré, Ambroise. *De la chirurgie.* In *Oeuvres.* 4th ed. Paris, 1585.

Percival, Thomas. *Medical Ethics: A Code of Institutions and Precepts Adapted to the Professional Conduct of Physicians and Surgeons.* Manchester, 1803 (1st ed., 1794).

Platina, Bartolomeo. *De honneste volupté.* Lyon, 1528.

Plato. *Opera omnia.* Translated by Ficino. Frankfurt, 1602.

———. *The Republic.* Ed. with English trans. by Paul Shorey. 2 vols. Loeb Classical Library. Cambridge, Mass., and London: Harvard University Press and Heinemann, 1963.

Platter, Felix. *Observationum libri tres.* Basel, 1614.

Pomis, David de. *De medico Hebraeo enarratio apologetica.* Venice, 1588.

Primrose, James. *De morbis mulierum.* Rotterdam, 1655.

Ranchin, François. *Opuscula medica.* Lyon, 1627.

Ricchieri, Ludovico (or Ludovicus Caelius Rhodoginus). *Lectionum antiquarum libri xxx.* Basel, 1542.

Rostinio, Pietro. *Trattato di mal francese.* Venice, 1556.

Rudio, Eustachio. *De morbis occultis et venenatis.* Venice, 1610. 1st ed., 1604.

Sanchez, Thomas. *Disputationes de sancto matrimonii sacramento.* 3 vols. Antwerp, 1607.

Santacruz, Alfonso Ponce de. *Dignotio et cura affectuum melancholicorum.* Madrid, 1622.

Sassonia, Ercole. *De melancholia.* Venice, 1620.

———. *Luis venereae perfectissimus tractatus.* Patavii, 1597.

Scaliger, Julius Caesar. *Exotericarum exercitationum liber XV de subtilitate.* Hannover, 1620.

Selvatico, Giovanni Battista. *De iis qui morbum simulant deprehendis.* Milan, 1595.

Sennert, Daniel. *Epitome institutionum medicinae.* Patavii, 1644.

———. *Opera omnia.* Lyon, 1666.

———. *Practica medica.* Paris, 1633.

————. Nicholas Culpeper, and Abdiah Cole. *Two Treatises. The First of the Venereal Pocks, The Second Treatise of the Gout.* London, 1660.

Sitoni, Giovanni Battista. *Miscellanea medico-curiosa.* 2d ed. Cologne, 1677.

Spach, Israel and Caspar Bauhin, eds. *Gynaeciorum sive de mulierum morbis.* Strassburg, 1597.

Textus Bibliae cum glossa ordinaria, Nicolai de Lyra Postilla . . . . Basel, 1508—?.

Torrella, Caspar. *Tractatus cum consiliis contra pudendagram seu morbum Gallicum.* Rome, 1497.

Valesius, Franciscus. *Controversiarum medicarum et philosophicarum.* 3d ed. Frankfurt, 1590.

Veiga, Tomás Rodriguez da. In *Claudii Galeni libros De locis affectis.* Antverp, 1566.

Vives, Juan Luis. *Opera.* Basel, 1555.

Whitney, Geoffrey. *A Choice of Emblemes.* Leiden, 1586.

Wither, George. *Britain's Remembrancer.* London, 1628.

Wolf, Hans Kaspar, ed. *Gynaeciorum, hoc est de mulierum tum aliis, tum gravidarum, parientium, et puerperarum affectibus et morbis, Libri veterum ac recentiorum.* Basel, 1566.

Zacchia, Paolo. *Quaestiones medico-legales.* Rome, 1634; 3d ed., Amsterdam, 1651.

Zacuto, Abraham. *De praxi medica libri tres.* Amsterdam, 1634.

————. *Opera omnia.* Lyon, 1642.

Zwinger, Theodor. *Theatrum humanae vitae.* Basel, 1604. (First ed. 1586–87.)

Secondary Sources

Alic, Margaret. *Hypatia's Heritage: A History of Women from Antiquity to the Late Nineteenth Century.* London: Women's Press, 1986.

Amundsen, Darrel W. "Casuistry and Professional Obligations: The Regulation of Physicians by the Court of Conscience in the Late Middle Ages." Pts. 1 and 2. *Transactions and Studies of the College of Physicians of Philadelphia,* 5th ser., vol. 3 (1981): 22–29, 93–112.

Baader, Gerhard. "Jacques Dubois as a Practitioner." In *The Medical Renaissance of the Sixteenth Century.* Ed. A. Wear, R. K. French, and I. M. Lonie. Cambridge: Cambridge University Press, 1985.

Bandeira, R. "La renaissance et l'Ecole Iatroéthique Portugaise du XVIe siècle." In *Atti, XXI Congresso internationale di Storia della Medicina (1988),* ed. Raffaele A. Bernabeo. Bologna: Monduzzi, 1988.

Boas, George. *The History of Ideas.* New York: Scribner's, 1969.

Bonner, Campbell. "The Trial of Saint Eugenia." *American Journal of Philology* 41 (1920): 260.

Brandt, Allan M. "The Syphilis Epidemic and Its Relationship to AIDS." *Science* 239 (1988): 375–80.

Castro, Américo. *The Spaniards: An Introduction to Their History.* Trans. W. F. King and S. Margaretten. Berkeley: University of California Press, 1971.

————. *The Structure of Spanish History.* Trans. E. L. King. Princeton, N.J.: Princeton University Press, 1954.

Crawford, Patricia. "Attitudes to Menstruation in Seventeenth-Century England." *Past and Present* 91 (1981): 47–73.

Culver, C. M., K. D. Clouser, B. Gert, et al. "Basic Curricular Goals in Medical Ethics." *New England Journal of Medicine* 312 (1985): 253–56.

Debus, Allen G. "Guintherius, Libavius and Sennert: The Chemical Compromise in Early Modern Medicine." In *Science, Medicine and Society in the Renaissance: Essays to Honor Walter Pagel.* Ed. Allen G. Debus. London: Heinemann, 1972.

DeMause, Lloyd. *The History of Childhood: The Untold Story of Child Abuse.* New York: Pedrick, 1988.

Derrida, Jacques. *La dissémination.* Paris: Seuil, 1972.

Diepgen, Paul. *Über den Einfluss der autoritativen Theologie auf die Medizin des Mittelalters.* Wiesbaden: Steiner, 1958.

Dizionario biográfico degli Italiani. Rome, 1960—.

Duerr, Hans Peter. *Der Mythos vom Zivilisationsprozess.* Vol. 1, *Nacktheit und Scham.* Frankfurt: Suhrkamp, 1988. Vol. 2, *Intimität.* Frankfurt: Suhrkamp, 1990.

Eccles, Audrey. *Obstetrics and Gynaecology in Tudor and Stuart England.* Kent, Ohio: Kent State University Press, 1982.

Eckart, Wolfgang-Uwe. "Grundlagen des medizinisch-wissenschaftlichen Erkennens bei Daniel Sennert (1572–1637) untersucht an seiner Schrift *De Chymicorum liber.*" M.D. diss., Universität Münster, 1978.

Elmer, Peter. "Medicine, Religion, and the Puritan Revolution." In *The Medical Revolution of the Seventeenth Century.* Ed. Roger French and Andrew Wear. Cambridge and New York: Cambridge University Press, 1989.

Encyclopedia of Bioethics. 4 vols. Ed. Warren T. Reich. London: Free Press, 1978.

Engelhardt, Dietrich von. "Geburt und Tod—medizinethische Betrachtungen in historischer Perspective." In *Anfang and Ende des menschlichen Lebens: Medizinethische Probleme.* Ed. O. Marquard and H. Staudinger. Paderborn: Schöningh, 1987.

————. "Medizinische Ethik in historischer Sicht." *Geriatrie und Rehabilitation* 3 (1990): 77–84.

————. "Medizinische Ethik in historischer Sicht: Renaissance, Aufklärung, Romantik." *Geriatrie und Rehabilitation* 3 (1990): 113–23.

Fabricius, Johannes. *Syphilis in Shakespeare's England.* London and Bristol, Pennsylvania: Jessica Kingsley, 1994.

Fee, Elizabeth. "Sin versus Science: Venereal Disease in 20th-Century Baltimore." In *AIDS: The Burdens of History.* Ed. Elizabeth Fee and Daniel M. Fox. Berkeley: University of California Press, 1988.

Feilchenfeld, Alfred. "Anfang und Blüthezeit der Portugiesengemeinde in Hamburg." *Zeitschrift für hamburgische Geschichte* 10 (1899): 199–240.

Figlio, Karl. "Chlorosis and Chronic Disease in 19th-Century Britain: The Social Construction of Somatic Illness in a Capitalist Society." In *Women and Health: The Politics of Sex in Medicine*. Ed. Elizabeth Fee. Farmingdale, N.Y.: Baywood, 1983.

Fineberg, Harvey V. "Education to Prevent AIDS: Prospects and Obstacles." *Science* 239 (1988): 592–96.

Foa, Anna. "The New and the Old: The Spread of Syphilis (1494–1530)." In *Sex and Gender in Historical Perspective: Selections from Quaderni Storici.* Ed. Edward Muir and Guido Ruggiero. Baltimore and London: Johns Hopkins University Press, 1990.

Friedenwald, Harry. *Jews and Medicine: Essays.* 2 vols. Baltimore: Johns Hopkins University Press, 1944.

———. "Montalto: A Jewish Physician at the Court of Marie de Medicis and Louis XIII." *Bulletin of the Institute of Historical Medicine* 3 (1935): 129–58.

Gilman, Sander, Helen King, Roy Porter, George Rousseau, and Elaine Showalter. *Hysteria Beyond Freud.* Berkeley and Los Angeles: University of California Press, 1993.

Gilman, Stephen. *The Spain of Fernando de Rojas: The Intellectual Landscape of La Celestina.* Princeton, N.J.: Princeton University Press, 1972.

Ginzburg, Carlo. *Il nicodemismo: Simulazione e dissimulazione religiosa nell'Europa del '500.* Torino: Einaudi, 1970.

Grafton, Anthony, with April Shelford, and Nancy Siraisi. *New Worlds, Ancient Texts: The Power of Tradition and the Shock of Discovery.* Cambridge, Mass.: Harvard University Press, 1992.

Green, Monica. "Women's Medical Practice and Health Care in Medieval Europe." *Signs* 14 (1989): 434–73.

Henry, John. "The Matter of Souls: Medical Theory and Theology in Seventeenth-Century England." In *The Medical Revolution of the Seventeenth Century.* Ed. Roger French and Andrew Wear. Cambridge: Cambridge University Press, 1989.

Hirsch, August. *Biographisches Lexikon der hervorragenden Ärzte aller Zeiten.* 2d ed. Berlin and Wien: Urban and Schwarzenberg, 1929–1932. 1st ed., 1883.

Historisches Wörterbuch der Philosophie. 6 vols. Basel und Stuttgart: Schwabe, 1971–[92].

Holcomb, Richmond Cranston. *Who Gave the World Syphilis? The Haitian Myth.* New York: Froben, 1937.

Homberger, E. Fischer. *Medizin vor Gericht: Gerichtsmedizin von der Renaissance bis zur Aufklärung.* Bern, Stuttgart, Wien: Huber, 1983.

Hsia, R. Po-Chia. *The Myth of Ritual Murder: Jews and Magic in Reformation Germany.* New Haven and London: Yale University Press, 1988.

Isler, M. "Zur ältesten Geschichte der Juden in Hamburg." *Zeitschrift für hamburgische Geschichte* 6 (1875): 461–79.

Israel, Jonathan I. *Empires and Entrepots: The Dutch, the Spanish Monarchy, and the Jews 1585–1713.* London and Roncevert, W.V.: Hambledon, 1990.

Jacquart, Danielle and Claude Thomasset. *Sexuality and Medicine in the Middle Ages.* Trans. Matthew Adamson. Princeton, N.J.: Princeton University Press, 1985.

Kant, Immanuel. *Werke.* Vol. 8. Frankfurt: Suhrkamp, 1968.

Kayserling, M. "Zur Geschichte der jüdischen Ärzte (II): Rodrigo a Castro." *Monatsschrift für Geschichte und Wissenschaft des Judenthums* 8 (1859): 330–39.

Kellenbenz, Herman. *Sephardim an der unteren Elbe: Ihre wirtschaftliche Bedeutung vom Ende des 16. bis zum Ende des 18. Jahrhunderts.* Wiesbaden: Franz Steiner, 1958.

Kibre, Pearl. *Hippocrates Latinus: Repertorium of Hippocratic Writings in the Latin Middle Ages.* Rev. ed. New York: Fordham University Press, 1985.

Der kranke Mensch in Mittelalter und Renaissasnce. Ed. Peter Wunderli. Forschungsinstitut für Mittelalter und Renaissance, Düsseldorf: Dorste, 1986.

Laqueur, Thomas. *Making Sex: Body and Gender from the Greeks to Freud.* Cambridge, Mass.: Harvard University Press, 1990.

Lemay, Helen R. "Anthonius Guainerius and Medieval Gynecology." In *Women of the Medieval World: Essays in Honor of John H. Munday.* Ed. Julius Kirshner and Suzanne F. Wemple. Oxford and New York: Blackwell, 1985.

Lewis, Bernard. *The Jews of Islam.* Princeton, N.J.: Princeton University Press, 1984.

MacDonald, Michael, ed. *Witchcraft and Hysteria in Elizabethan London: Edward Jorden and the Mary Glover Case.* London and New York: Tavistock/Routledge, 1991.

Maclean, Ian. *The Renaissance Notion of Woman: A Study in the Fortunes of Scholasticism and Medieval Science in European Intellectual Life.* Cambridge: Cambridge University Press, 1985.

Matuschka, M. E., Graf. "Ärztliche Deontologie im Mittelalter." *Die medizinische Welt* 37 (1986): 378–80.

Morejón, Antonio Hernández. *Historia bibliográfica de la medicina española.* 7 vols. Madrid, 1842–52.

Muir, Edward and Guido Ruggiero, eds. *Sex and Gender in Historical Perspective: Selections from Quaderni Storici.* Baltimore and London: Johns Hopkins University Press, 1990.

Nagy, Gregory. *The Best of the Achaeans: Concepts of the Hero in Archaic Greek Poetry.* Baltimore and London: Johns Hopkins University Press, 1979.

Niccoli, Ottavia. "'Menstruum Quasi Monstrum': Monstrous Births and Menstrual Taboo in the Sixteenth Century." In Muir and Ruggiero, eds., *Sex and Gender in Historical Perspective.*

Niebyl, Peter H. "Sennert, Van Helmont and Medical Ontology." *Bulletin of the History of Medicine* 45 (1971): 115–37.

Niewoehner, Friedrich. *Veritas sive varietas: Lessings Toleranzparabel und das Buch Von den drei Betrügern.* Heidelberg: Lambert Schneider, 1988.

Noonan, John T. *Contraception: A History of Its Treatment by the Catholic Theologians and Canonists.* Cambridge, Mass.: Harvard University Press, 1986.

Noreña, Carlos C. *Juan Luis Vives.* International Archives of the History of Ideas, no. 34. The Hague: Nijhoff, 1970.

Oppenheimer, Gerald M. "In the Eye of the Storm: The Epidemiological Construction of AIDS." In *AIDS: The Burden of History*. Ed. Elizabeth Fee and Daniel M. Fox. Berkeley: University of California Press, 1988.

"Popes." In *Encyclopaedia Judaica*. Jerusalem: Keter, 1972–82.

Quétel, Claude. *History of Syphilis*. Trans. J. Braddock and Brian Pike. London: Polity Press, 1990.

Read, Conyers. *Mr. Secretary Cecil and Queen Elizabeth*. London: Cape, 1962.

Reed, Malcolm K. *Juan Huarte de San Juan*. Boston: Twayne, 1981.

Rosebury, Theodor. *Microbes and Morals: The Strange Story of Venereal Disease*. New York: Viking, 1971.

Roth, Cecil. *A History of the Marranos*. Philadelphia: The Jewish Publication Society of America, 1947.

Ruderman, David B. *Kabbalah, Magic, and Science: The Cultural Universe of a Sixteenth-Century Jewish Physician*. Cambridge, Mass.: Harvard University Press, 1988.

———. *A Valley of Vision: The Heavenly Journey of Abraham Yagel*. Philadelphia: University of Pennsylvania Press, 1990.

Sanwald, Erich. *Otto Brunfels 1488–1535: Ein Beitrag zur Geschichte des Humanismus und der Reformation* Diss. München. Bottrop: Postberg, 1932.

Schadewaldt, Hans. "Arzt und Patient in antiker und frühchristlicher Sicht." *Medizinische Klinik* 59 (1964): 146–52.

Schleiner, Winfried. "Burton's Use of *praeteritio* in Discussing Same-Sex Relationships." In *Renaissance Discourses of Desire*. Ed. C. J. Summers and T. L. Pebworth. Columbia, Mo., and London: University of Missouri Press, 1993.

———. *The Imagery of John Donne's Sermons*. Providence, R.I.: Brown University Press, 1970.

———. "Infection and Cure through Women: Renaissance Constructions of Syphilis." *Journal of Medieval and Renaissance Studies* 24 (1994): 501–17.

———. "Justifying the Unjustifiable: The Dover Cliff Scene in *King Lear*." *Shakespeare Quarterly* 36 (1985): 337–43.

———. "Le feu caché: Homosocial Bonds Between Women in a Renaissance Romance." *Renaissance Quarterly* 45 (1992): 293–311.

———. *Melancholy, Genius, and Utopia in the Renaissance*. Wolfenbütteler Abhandlungen zur Renaissanceforschung, 10. Wiesbaden: Harrassowitz, 1991.

———. "Renaissance Exempla of Schizophrenia: The Cure by Charity in Luther and Cervantes." *Renaissance and Reformation* 9 (1985): 157–76.

———. The Contribution of Exiled Portuguese Jews in "Renaissance Medical Ethics." In *Expulsion of the Jews: 1492 and After*. Ed. R. B. Waddington and A. H. Williamson. New York and London: Garland, 1994.

———. "Renaissance Moralizing of Syphilis and Moral Issues about Prevention." *Bulletin of the History of Medicine* 68 (1994): 389–410.

———. "'That Matter Which Ought Not To Be Heard Of': Homophobic Slurs in Renaissance Cultural Politics." *Journal of Homosexuality* 26 (1994): 41–75.

Schmitt, Charles B. *The Aristotelian Tradition and Renaissance Universities.* London: Variorum Reprints, 1984.

Schröder, Hans. *Lexikon der hamburgischen Schriftsteller.* Hamburg, 1851.

Showalter, Elaine. *The Female Malady: Women, Madness, and English Culture 1830–1980.* New York: Pantheon, 1985.

Siraisi, Nancy G. *Avicenna in Renaissance Italy: The Canon and Medical Teaching in Italian Universities after 1500.* Princeton, N.J.: Princeton University Press, 1987.

———. *Taddeo Alderotti and his Pupils: Two Generations of Italian Medical Learning.* Princeton, N.J.: Princeton University Press, 1981.

Smith, Bruce R. *Homosexual Desire in Shakespeare's England: A Cultural Poetics.* Chicago and London: University of Chicago Press, 1991.

Smith, Wesley D. *The Hippocratic Tradition.* Ithaca, N.Y., Cornell University Press, 1979.

Spira, Moses A. "Meilensteine der jüdischen Ärzte in Deutschland." In *Melemata: Festschrift für Werner Leibbrand.* Ed. Joseph Schumacher, Martin Schrenk, and Jörn H. Wolf. Mannheim: Mannheimer Grossdruckerei, 1967.

Sudhoff, Karl, and Charles Singer. *The Earliest Printed Literature on Syphilis.* Florence: Lier, 1925.

Temkin, Owsei. *The Double Face of Janus and Other Essays in the History of Medicine.* Baltimore and London: Johns Hopkins University Press, 1977.

———. *Galenism: Rise and Decline of a Medical Philosophy.* Ithaca, N.Y.: Cornell University Press, 1973.

———. *Hippocrates in a World of Pagans and Christians.* Baltimore and London: Johns Hopkins University Press, 1991.

Veith, Ilza. *Hysteria: The History of a Disease.* Chicago and London: University of Chicago Press, 1965.

Vickers, Brian, ed. *Occult and Scientific Mentalities in the Renaissance.* Cambridge: Cambridge University Press, 1984.

Weinrich, Harald. *Das Ingenium Don Quijotes.* Forschungen zur Romanischen Philologie, Heft 1. Münster: Aschendorf, 1956.

Whaley, Joachim. *Religious Toleration and Social Change in Hamburg, 1529–1819.* Cambridge: Cambridge University Press, 1985.

Williams, Neville. *Thomas Howard, Fourth Duke of Norfolk.* London: Barrie and Rockliff, 1964.

Yerushalmi, Yoseph Hayim. *From Spanish Court to Italian Ghetto: Isaac Cardoso; A Study in Seventeenth-Century Marranism and Jewish Apologetics.* New York and London: Columbia University Press, 1971.

Zagorin, Perez. *Ways of Lying: Dissimulation, Persecution, and Conformity in Early Modern Europe.* Cambridge, Mass., and London: Harvard University Press, 1990.

Index

Abortion: ethics of, 5, 28, 34, 35–37, 42; of dead foetus as compared to removal of female seed, 123

Adstantes ("persons standing by" the patient's bed; the world immediately surrounding it), 7–8, 40, 42; as moral arbiters, 36; physician's duty to inform, 31, 32; role in cure of patient, 29–37

Aelianus, 11

Agatha, Saint, 20

Agnodice (Hagnodice), 18–19, 40

Agrippa, Cornelius, 24

AIDS: and social construction of disease, 183; as related to syphilis, 195, 199 n.39, 208; prevention of, x, 208

Albi, Johannes Rodericus Castelli (Amatus Lusitanus), 61, 78–80, 82, 118, 119

Alciati, 188

Alderotti, Taddeo, 24

Alessandrini, Julius (Alexandrinus), ix, 20, 26, 42, 46 n.45, 74–78, 203, 206

Alic, Margaret, 44 n.30

Almenar, Juan, 169

Alzaharavius (Albukasis), 132

Amatus Lusitanus. *See* Albi.

Ambrose, 57

Amundsen, Darrel W., vii, 43 n.13, 105 n.7

Antidote (or "mullet"), against syphilis infection, 178, 179, 181

Anti-Jewish propaganda, 81–83, 94, 125, 206

Antoninus of Florence, 67

Aquinas, Thomas, 1

Arcediano, 66

Argenterio, Giovanni, 14, 46 n.45

Aristotle, 6, 11, 12, 42, 43 n.12, 57, 59, 75, 95, 108, 109, 110, 127, 145; *Nichomachean Ethics*, xi n.1, 1, 145

Aristotelian natural philosophy, vii, 25

Arnald of Villanova, 31

Attendolo, Iacobo Francisco, 193

Augustine, Saint, 44 n.18

Augustinus of Ancona, 67

Autosuggestion, use of in treatment, 25, 204

Avicenna, 25, 26, 81, 113, 125, 135, 148, 149

Avila, Louis Lobera d', 35

Azor, Juan, 35

Baader, Gerhard, 153 n.9

Bacon, Francis, 8, 61

Bandeira, R., 202 n.70

Bardi, Girolamo, ix, 19, 94–97, 195, 204

Barrough, Philip, 112, 163–166, 167, 170, 183

Bartholin, Thomas, 159 n.76

Bauhin, 119

Benaker, Jacob, 83

Bible: New Testament, 1, 2, 11; Old Testament, 2, 10, 12, 27, 29, 57, 58–59, 71, 95, 109–110, 134

Black (or African) women, coition with to cure syphilis, 189–190, 191

221

£15·75

ıurn by.
ıate below

——— ..